ENDOSCOPIC PARANASAL SINUS SURGERY

Chapter 3 contributed by

Terry S. Becker, M.D.

Associate Professor of Clinical Radiology
University of Southern California
L.A.C.-U.S.C. Medical Center
Los Angeles, California

Barbara Zeifer Ukra, M.D.

Instructor of Radiology
University of Southern California
L.A.C.-U.S.C. Medical Center
Los Angeles, California

ENDOSCOPIC PARANASAL SINUS SURGERY

Dale H. Rice, M.D.

Tiber/Alpert Professor and Chairman
Department of Otolaryngology—Head and Neck Surgery
University of Southern California School of Medicine
Los Angeles, California

Steven D. Schaefer, M.D.

Professor, Chairman, Division of Head and Neck Surgery
Department of Otorhinolaryngology
University of Texas Southwestern Medical Center
Dallas, Texas

with illustrations by

Lewis E. Calver

Associate Professor
Biomedical Communications
University of Texas Southwestern Medical Center
Dallas, Texas

Raven Press 🦅 New York

Raven Press, 1185 Avenue of the Americas, New York, New York 10036

Made in the United States of America

Library of Congress Cataloging−in−Publication Data

Rice, Dale H.
    Endoscopic paranasal sinus surgery / Dale H. Rice, Steven D.
Schaefer ; with illustrations by Lewis E. Calver.
       p.   cm.
    Includes bibliographies and index.
    ISBN 0-88167-473-7
    1. Paranasal sinuses—Surgery—Atlases. 2. Endoscopic surgery—
-Atlases. I. Schaefer, Steven D., 1945–   II. Title.
    [DNLM: 1. Endoscopy—atlases. 2. Paranasal Sinuses—surgery
atlases. WV 17 R495e]
RF421.R48 1988
617′.51—dc19
DNLM/DLC
for Library of Congress   88−18498
                                                       CIP

9 8 7 6 5 4 3 2 1

Cover illustration by Lewis E. Calver

*To our wives Barbara and Phyllis
and our children Alexander and Jessica*

PREFACE

Several years ago, we had the good fortune to be instructed thoroughly in the Messerklinger and Wigand techniques of endoscopic sinus surgery. Despite the polarity in Europe, it became clear with experience, that the differences were more imagined than real and that both techniques had their appropriate uses. Since then, we have had extensive personal experience using these techniques with patients, and numerous opportunities to teach them at lectures and courses.

The purpose of this book is to provide a reference atlas for the rhinologic surgeon. It is not to teach the Messerklinger and Wigand techniques. For anyone who wishes to learn endoscopic sinus surgery, we strongly advise (1) to first attend a course that includes cadaver dissections; then (2) purchase the equipment necessary for the clinical examination of patients; and (3) continue to perform conventional sinus surgery, but examine the operative site with the endoscopes before, during, and after the procedure. Such examination will allow further familiarization with the usefulness of the endoscopes and with the anatomy of the area. Finally (4) one can then begin to perform endoscopic sinus surgery when comfortable with the instruments and the anatomy.

Dale H. Rice
Steven D. Schaefer

CONTENTS

ENDOSCOPIC PARANASAL SINUS SURGERY

Introduction

There is no new thing under the sun.
—Ecclesiastes 1:9

Hirschmann in 1901 used a modified cystoscope to examine the sinuses (Draf, 1983). The current interest in endoscopic sinus surgery stems from several developments. First has been the advent of compact, multiangled telescopes that allow excellent visualization of the nasal cavity for examination and of the sinuses during procedures, including such areas as the maxillary ostium and the frontal recess. Second has been the acceptance and appreciation of the great work of Messerklinger demonstrating that the anterior ethmoids usually are the key to persistent sinusitis (Messerklinger, 1967). Third has been the CT scan. The CT scan has shown clearly what plain roentgenograms and complex motion tomography could not—that the anterior ethmoids are usually diseased when the condition would appear to be only maxillary or frontal sinusitis. These developments make it possible to diagnose more accurately and treat sinusitis refractory to noninvasive therapy.

The techniques of endoscopic sinus surgery were developed in Europe by Messerklinger and Wigand, who had two different goals. For nonmedical reasons, there has been some polarization of the proponents of these two techniques, when, in fact, they are designed for different extremes of disease, and there is considerable blurring of the distinctions for intermediate disease. The Messerklinger technique (1985) is ideal for the patient with anterior ethmoid disease with or without maxillary or frontal sinus disease. The Wigand technique (1978), in contrast, is ideal for the patient with pansinusitis who has or is apt to fail the more limited Messerklinger approach.

Both techniques are based on the assumption that the sinus mucosa is most likely reversibly diseased and will return to normal once adequate drainage has been established. Interestingly, this return to normal seems to occur clinically but has not been demonstrated histologically. No attempt is made to eradicate the sinus mucous membrane, as in the Caldwell-Luc procedure, but rather to reestablish drainage so the mucosa can return to normal and resume its proper function.

The Messerklinger technique is an anterior-to-posterior approach that most commonly involves only the anterior ethmoids and the maxillary sinus ostium. Bear in mind that it can be extended into the posterior ethmoids, sphenoid, and frontal sinuses if necessary. The Wigand approach is posterior-to-anterior and routinely involves all the sinuses on the involved side. Thus, the technique used should fit the disease.

LITERATURE CITED

Draf, W.
  1983 *Endoscopy of the Paranasal Sinuses.* Springer-Verlag, New York.
Messerklinger, W.
  1985 Endoskopische Diagnose und Chirurgie der rezidivierenden Sinusitis. In: *Advances in Nose and Sinus Surgery,* edited by Z. Krajina. Zagreb University, Zagreb, Yugoslavia.
Messerklinger, W.
  1967 Uber die Drainage der Menschlichen Nasennebenhohler unter normalen und pathologischen Bendingunger. II. Mitterlung: Die Stirnhohle und ihr Ausfuhrungssystem. *Monatsschr. Ohrenheilhd.,* 101:313–326.
Wigand, M. E., Steiner, W., and Jaumann, M. P.
  1978 Endonasal sinus surgery with endoscopical control: From radical operation to rehabilitation of the mucosa. *Endoscopy,* 10:255–260.

1

Anatomy of the Paranasal Sinuses

The paranasal sinuses are among the most poorly described anatomic sites in the human body because of the great variations within individuals and the inconsistency of terminology in describing these structures. The problems in terminology arose from initial confusion about the origin of individual sinuses and the active debate among surgeons in the first half of the twentieth century about the treatment of acute and chronic sinusitis (Blanton and Biggs, 1969). In this preantibiotic era, much attention was directed toward anatomic studies justifying either cannulation or puncture of the sinuses (Myerson, 1932; Van Alyea, 1936; Simon, 1939; Rosenberger, 1938; Kasper, 1936; Schaeffer, 1916). From this era came a consensus that the sinuses could be understood best by study of their embryology, and from that consensus came the foundations of modern sinus surgery. In the context of endoscopic sinus surgery, the importance of treating ethmoid disease as a source of recurrent frontal or maxillary sinusitis was recognized as early as 1916, when J. Parsons Schaeffer stated that "the maxillary sinus is often a cesspool for infectious material from the sinus frontalis and certain of the anterior group of cellulae ethmoidales" (Schaeffer, 1916). Such is an example of knowledge lost, only to be rediscovered when new interest in the sinuses arose following advances in instrument technology and the work of modern sinus surgeons (Messerklinger, 1985; Wigand et al., 1978).

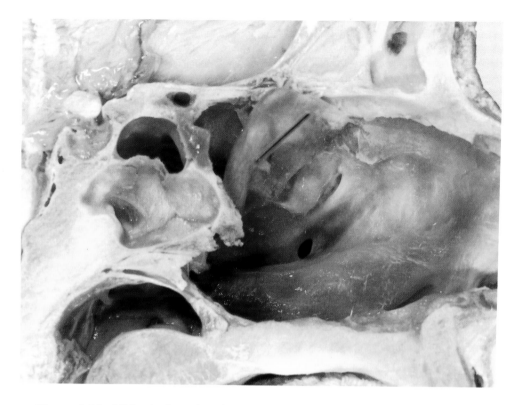

Figure 1.1A. Midsagittal section showing anatomy of the lateral nasal wall. Middle turbinate has been deflected superiorly to reveal the surface anatomy of the ethmoid sinus.

ETHMOID SINUS

Embryology and Development (Figures 1.1–1.8)

Of all the paranasal sinuses, the ethmoid sinus has the greatest variation, and it is best understood by reviewing its embryologic development. The anterior cells of this sinus first appear in the third fetal month as evaginations (also termed "pits" or "furrows") of the lateral nasal wall adjacent to the middle meatus (Kasper, 1936). The origin of these pits is the frontal recess, which in turn originates from the middle meatus. In the coronal plane, these pits can be likened to troughs in a wave, with the peaks represented by thickened cartilage that later will become the turbinates or nasal concha. The uncinate process and bulla ethmoidalis can be considered accessory peaks or, more correctly, folds, and the ethmoidal infundibulum and suprabullar furrow as accessory pits (Kasper, 1936; Libersa et al., 1981).

At birth, the anterior (or anteromiddle cells, depending on the division of the sinus into two or three parts) ethmoid sinus measures $2 \times 2 \times 5$ mm, and the posterior sinus measures $2 \times 4 \times 5$ mm. At this time, the ethmoids are fluid-filled and are difficult to recognize on routine radiography. They may be consistently visualized by this form of x-ray only at age 1 year and then

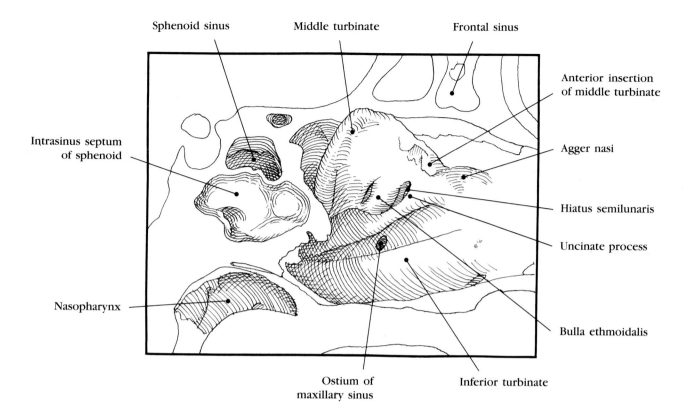

Sphenoid sinus   Middle turbinate   Frontal sinus

Anterior insertion
of middle turbinate

Intrasinus septum
of sphenoid

Agger nasi

Hiatus semilunaris

Uncinate process

Nasopharynx

Bulla ethmoidalis

Ostium of
maxillary sinus   Inferior turbinate

Figure 1.1B. The hiatus semilunaris appears as a depression between the bulla ethmoidalis and the uncinate process. Anterior to the uncinate ridge is the agger nasi, which is formed by the pneumatization of the lacrimal bone by the infundibular cells of the ethmoid.

only if they are well developed (Shapiro and Janzen, 1960). As the ethmoid cells invade or pneumatize adjacent bones over the subsequent decade, the resultant sinuses may be named by the bone containing them rather than by their cell of origin (Figures 1.1, 1.3, 6.2C). Thus, an anterior ethmoid cell giving rise to a cavity within the frontal bone is known as the "frontal sinus." By the 12th year, the ethmoids have reached nearly adult size, with expansion during puberty primarily involving bones outside the ethmoid capsule (Van Alyea, 1951).

Clinical Anatomy

In the adult, the ethmoid sinuses form a pyramid, the wider base being located posteriorly and the entire sinus measuring 4 cm to 5 cm anteroposterior, 2.5 cm in height, and 0.5 cm wide anteriorly and 1.5 cm posteriorly (Mosher, 1929). The roof of the sinus, the **fovea ethmoidalis**, extends 2 mm to 3 mm above the more medial cribriform plate. The lateral wall is **the lamina papyracea (orbital plate)**, which forms the most constant part of the sinus (Figures 1.6, 1.7). The actual reported size of the sinus and the number of cells vary with each series, with one investigator examining 100

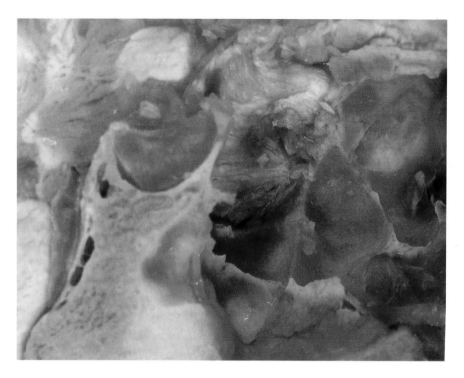

Figure 1.2A. Parasagittal section through the sphenoid and posterior ethmoid sinuses. The lateral wall of these sinuses has been removed to expose the cavernous sinus and optic nerve.

specimens and reporting a range of 4 to 17 cells per specimen, with an average of 9 cells (Van Alyea, 1939). The fact that the sinus is known as the "ethmoid labyrinth" attests to the intricacy of the structure and challenges our understanding of the anatomy.

For this discussion, cells are divided into those that are within the ethmoid capsule, or intramural, and those that are outside the ethmoid, or extramural. The intramural cells are further divided into the smaller but more numerous anterior cells and the larger posterior cells, with some authors calling the ethmoid bulla "middle cells" (Figure 1.3). The anterior ethmoid cells can be placed into subgroups on the basis of their location or that of their ostia (Van Alyea, 1939). However, cells of a given origin frequently invade the territory usually occupied by cells of another origin, and at least one author favors classification by the location of their ostia (Hollingshead, 1968). Examples of several classifications are shown in Table 1.1.

Of these classifications, and others not shown, the Ritter nomenclature conveys most clearly the origin and drainage of the ethmoid cells. Using Ritter's classification, the most anterior cells are the **frontal recess** cells (range 0–4 cells), which arise from the anterosuperior growth of the ethmoid into

Pituitary   Cavernous sinus   Optic nerve

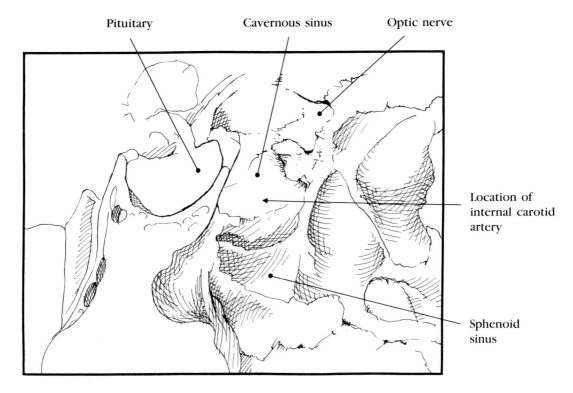

Location of
internal carotid
artery

Sphenoid
sinus

Figure 1.2B. The proximity of the optic nerve and internal carotid artery to the lateral wall of the sphenoid and posterior ethmoid sinuses is illustrated.

TABLE 1.1. *Classification of sinus cells*

Middle meatus	Anterior ethmoid cells	Anterior ethmoid cells
Infundibular cells	Frontal recess	Frontal recess
Agger nasi	Infundibular	Infundibular
Terminal	Bullar	Bullar (middle)
Suprainfundibular	Conchal	Conchal
Inferior	Extramural (i.e.,	Extramural
Bullar	agger nasi)	**Posterior ethmoid cells**
Bullar	**Posterior ethmoid cells**	Intramural
Suprabullar	Intramural	Extramural
Superior meatus	Extramural	*(Hollingshead, 1968)*
Posterior cells	*(Ritter, 1978)*	
Supreme meatus		
Postreme cells		
(Van Alyea, 1939)		

7

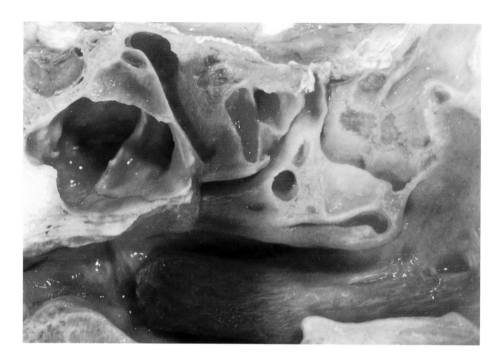

Figure 1.3A. Parasagittal section through the middle turbinate is shown.

the frontal bone (Figure 1.4). These cells may come to rest within the frontal bone, forming the frontal sinus, or give rise to a bulla or bulge into the frontal sinus floor, or form the supraorbital ethmoid cells as they pneumatize the orbit (Ritter, 1978). The inferior expansion of these cells can displace the nasofrontal duct, resulting in a serpentine course of the duct.

The **infundibular** cells (range 1–7 cells) are the next most anterior cells (Figure 1.5). The most constant of these cells are those that form the extramural cells, the **agger nasi**, through the pneumatization of the lacrimal bone (Van Alyea, 1939). These cells are located on the lateral nasal wall immediately anterior to the middle turbinate and are an important landmark in both intranasal procedures and external ethmoidectomy, since they are the cells first entered in these operations. They drain into the **ethmoid infundibulum**, which is a pouch or trough that ends superiorly in the **frontal recess**, and in some people, these cells may be the origin of the frontal sinus (Schaeffer, 1916) (Figure 1.1).

The **bullar** cells (range 1–6 cells) are the most constant of the anterior ethmoid cells and form a partial sphere lateral or beneath the middle turbinate, the **bulla ethmoidalis** (Van Alyea, 1939) (Figures 1.1, 1.3, 1.7). These cells drain into the middle meatus via crescentic ostia that lie superiorly, posteriorly, and parallel to the much larger semilunar cleft in the lateral nasal wall, the hiatus semilunaris (Van Alyea, 1939; Schaeffer, 1916). The **hiatus semilunaris** forms the curved groove between the bulla ethmoidalis, which borders it posteriorly, and its anterior border, which is a ridge of

Sphenoethmoid recess

Frontal
recess

Sphenoid
sinus

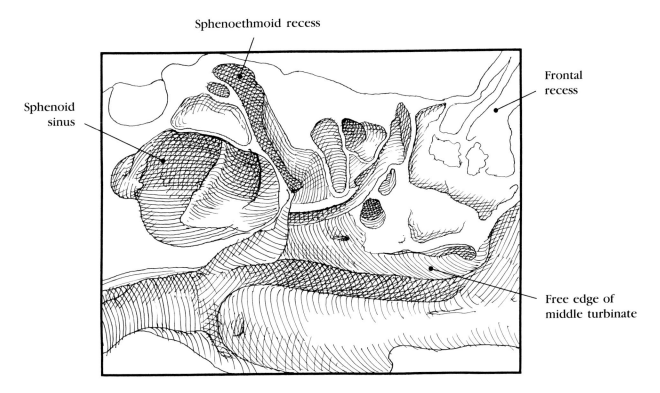

Free edge of
middle turbinate

Figure 1.3B. Extensive pneumatization of the ethmoid bone is shown, as represented by the anterior and posterior ethmoid sinuses.

bone formed by the ascending process of the maxilla, the uncinate process (Mosher, 1929) (Figure 1.1). Superiorly, the hiatus communicates with the ethmoid infundibulum. As the anterior boundary of the hiatus semilunaris, the **uncinate process** also is a semilunar structure, which ranges from nearly flat to 4 mm in height or projection into the nasal cavity and 14 mm to 22 mm in length (Myerson, 1932) (Figures 1.1, 5.2A, 6.2A). The uncinate process is immediately posterior to the agger nasi cells and, therefore, may or may not be visualized easily on the lateral nasal wall, depending on the anterior and inferior expansion of the middle turbinate.

Some authors prefer to divide the hiatus semilunaris into anterior and posterior portions, whereas others tend to describe it as extending from the superior terminal of the frontal recess to the posterior aspect of the bulla, thus either including or substituting the anterosuperior portion of the hiatus for part of the ethmoid infundibulum. Others consider the infundibulum to be the bottom or most lateral region of hiatus, describing the anterosuperior aspect as the ethmoid infundibulum (e.g., frontal recess to the bulla ethmoidalis) and designating the part of the infundibulum that communicates with the natural ostium of the maxillary sinus as the maxillary infundibulum (Mosher, 1929; Myerson, 1932). Whatever terminology is used, these structures are important landmarks and constitute the route by which secretions can flow from the frontal and anterior ethmoid cells into the ostium of the maxillary sinus (Schaeffer, 1916). On the medial, superior surface of the bulla is a furrow, the **suprabullar furrow**, that can evaginate to form **su-**

1.4A

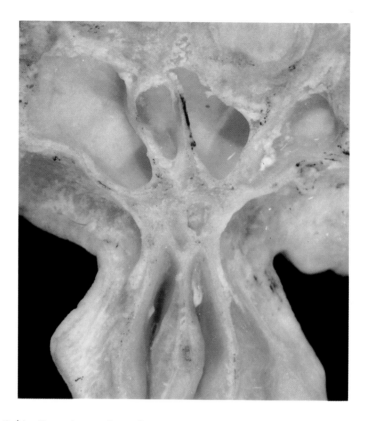

Figure 1.4A. Posterior surface of coronal section at the ventral aspect of the frontal sinus is shown.

Figure 1.4B. This section is sufficiently ventral to the body of the frontal sinus to include only a remnant of the frontal recess or the frontal recess cells of the anterior ethmoid.

Figure 1.4C. Plain film radiograph of the specimen shown in Figure 1.4A.

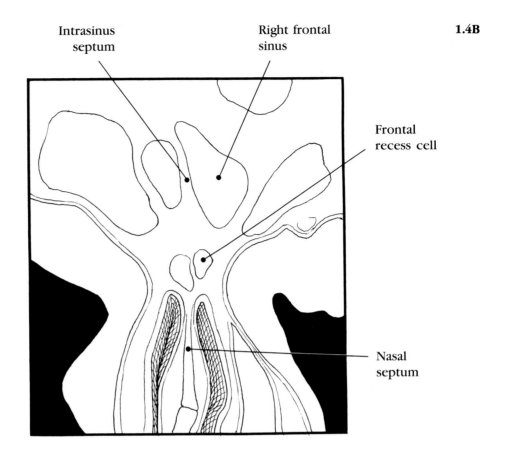

Intrasinus septum

Right frontal sinus

1.4B

Frontal recess cell

Nasal septum

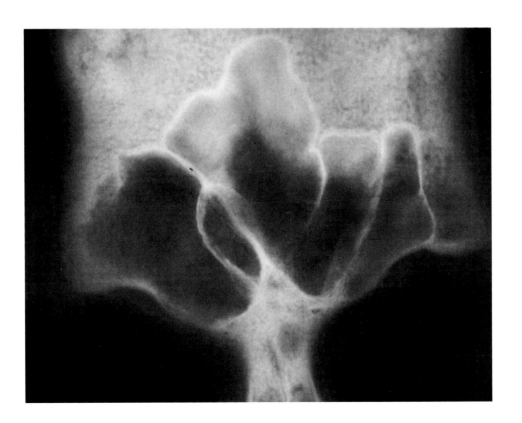

1.4C

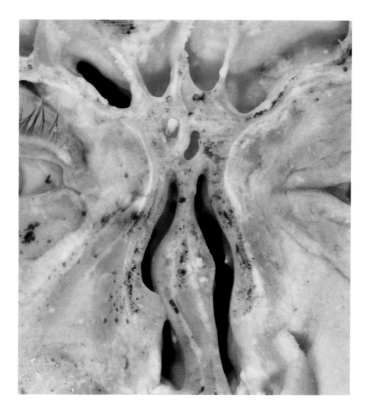

Figure 1.5A. Anterior surface of coronal section through frontal sinus contiguous with section in Figure 1.4A is shown.

prabullar cells within the ethmoid and adjacent bones.

The **conchal** cells invade the middle turbinate, and when these cells are located in the anterior aspect of the turbinate, they are referred to as a **"concha bullosa"** (Schaeffer, 1910a; Zuckerlandl, 1893) (Figures 1.3, 5.12A). The bullosa cells are clinically important because they can be an isolated source of recurrent ethmoiditis, or they may obstruct the middle meatus. The **middle turbinate** is the medial appendage of the nasal wall and overhangs the bulla ethmoidalis, hiatus semilunaris, and uncinate process (Figure 6.2). However, occasionally both the uncinate process and hiatus semilunaris are not covered by the downward expansion of this 3.5 cm to 4 cm long important bony landmark. Anteriorly, the middle turbinate is attached superiorly to the cribriform plate, with its free margin sloping posteroinferiorly 15 degrees so that the posterior tip lies at or immediately inferior to the sphenopalatine foramen (Ritter, 1978).

Major attachment for the middle turbinate to the ethmoid capsule and lamina papyracea is formed by ground plates or lamella. The most important of these, the **grand** or **basal lamella**, separates the anterior ethmoids from the posterior ethmoids (Zuckerkandl, 1893) (Figure 5.6A). Other lamella help to compartmentalize the ethmoid and may offer a brief barrier to the spread of infection.

Frontal recess cell

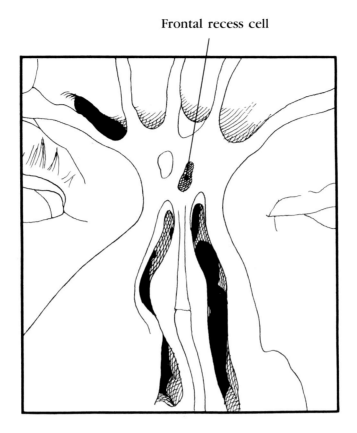

Figure 1.5B. Note frontal recess cells seen in the coronal section in Figure 1.5A. These cells are among the several possible origins of the frontal sinus.

The **posterior ethmoid** cells (range 1–7 cells) not only invade the posterior ethmoid capsule but also may involve the middle turbinate and the sphenoid, palatine, and maxillary bones (Figures 1.3, 1.7, 1.8). At the junction of the lamina papyracea and the frontal bone, the posterior ethmoidal artery enters the posterior ethmoids approximately 3 mm to 8 mm (average 5 mm) anterior to the optic nerve. In rare cases, the optic nerve may be surrounded by posterior extramural ethmoid cells. Both the anterior and posterior ethmoidal arteries lie at the articulation of the lamella of the middle and superior turbinate with the lamina papyracea (Ritter, 1978).

FRONTAL SINUS

Embryology and Development (Figures 1.1, 1.3, 1.4, 1.5)

The frontal sinus has several possible origins, each of which influences the relationship of this sinus to the lateral nasal wall, particularly the embryologic anterosuperior extension of the middle meatus, the **frontal recess** (Figures 1.1, 1.4, 1.5). Development of the frontal sinus is initiated in the fourth fetal month, when the entire nasofrontal area is represented by the frontal recess. Each frontal sinus may have a different origin and a unique

1.5C

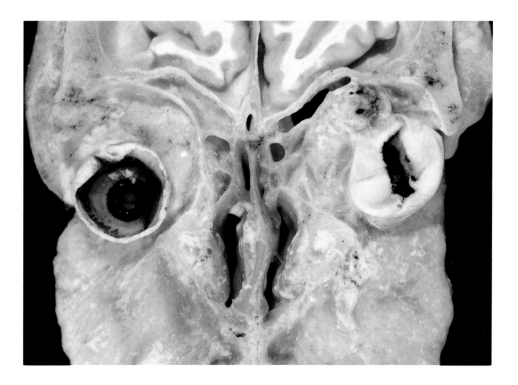

Figure 1.5C. Posterior surface of specimen in Figure 1.5A is sectioned immediately dorsal to the principal cavity of the frontal sinus.

Figure 1.5D. Supraorbital ethmoid cells are shown immediately superior to infundibular cells of the anterior ethmoid. The lateral boundary of these cells is the lamina papyracea, which is the most constant structure in the ethmoid bone.

Figure 1.5E. Plain film radiograph of the specimen shown in Figures 1.5A, C.

1.5D

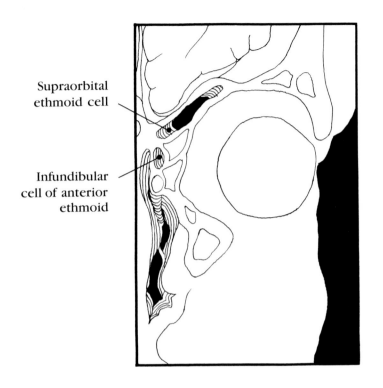

Supraorbital
ethmoid cell

Infundibular
cell of anterior
ethmoid

1.5E

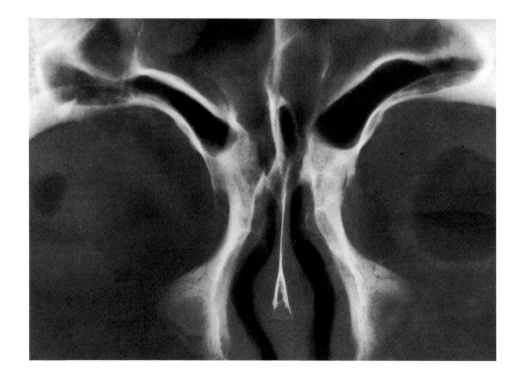

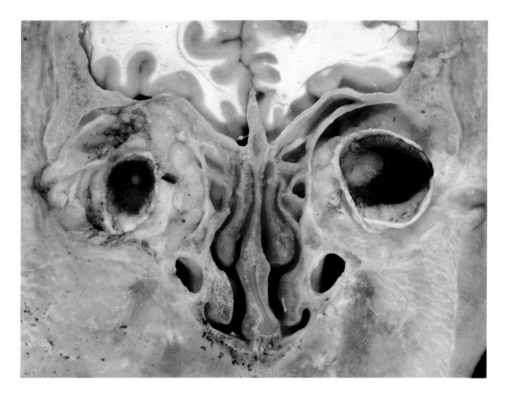

Figure 1.6A. The anterior surface of the coronal section contiguous with Figure 1.5C is shown. It is at the level of the ventral aspect of the maxillary sinus.

communication within the middle meatus. In a study of 100 adult specimens, Kasper found the most common origin of the frontal sinus to be pits or furrows in the frontal recess that were rudimentary anterior ethmoid cells (described previously as frontal recess cells). The more remote or lateral these pits are from the ethmoid infundibulum, the more lateral are the frontal sinus and its communication with the nose (Kasper, 1936). Kasper found that in more than 50% of the specimens, a sound placed in the ethmoid infundibulum would not pass freely into the frontal sinus. When the sinus arises from the ethmoid infundibular cells, the connection with the nose tends to be more in alignment with the ethmoid infundibulum. Far less common is the frontal sinus that is derived from direct extension of the entire frontal recess. In such a case, the communication "between the frontal sinus and the middle meatus can be expected to be large and roomy" (Kasper, 1936), depending on the impinging anterior ethmoid cells. At birth, the sinus has little clinical relevance, often being indistinguishable from the anterior ethmoid cells. By age 12 years, the frontal sinus is still somewhat smaller than adult size, with growth being completed before age 20 years (Van Alyea, 1951).

Cribriform plate   Crista galli   Supraorbital ethmoid cell

Infundibular cells of ethmoid

Middle turbinate

Maxillary sinus

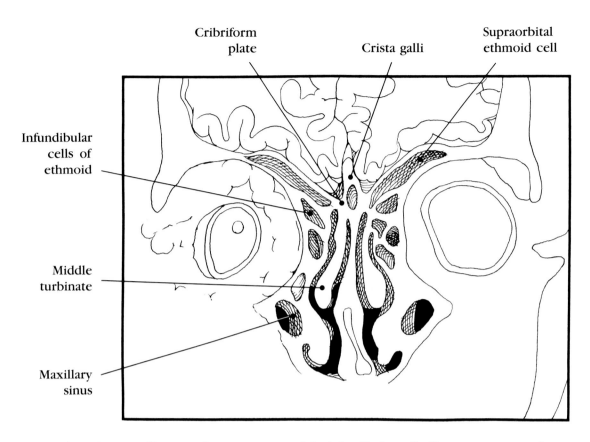

Figure 1.6B. Note the continuation of the infundibular cells. The most constant of these cells is the agger nasi, or pneumatization of the lacrimal bone.

Clinical Anatomy

The adult frontal sinus is described as measuring 28 mm high, 24 mm wide, and 20 mm deep (Schaeffer, 1920). This ideal sinus is a representative average, with the actual size and configuration reflecting the origin of the cavity and superior development into the squama of the frontal bone (Hollingshead, 1968). The sinus is compartmentalized further by intrasinus septa and marginated by irregular bone. The absence of the scalloped border or the intrasinus septa on plain film radiographs indicates significant infection (Wigh, 1950). The communication of this sinus with the nose usually is described as a distinct nasofrontal duct. More often, this is not the case, with the sinus instead draining by an ostium that, in the authors' experience, can vary from 2 mm to 10 mm in size (average <5 mm). As stated previously, this connection with the nose may drain either directly to the frontal recess or through the anterior ethmoid cells. There is significant variability in the accessibility of this passage via the nose, depending on the origin of this sinus from the frontal recess, anterior ethmoid cells, or ethmoid infundibulum (Van Alyea, 1941; Van Alyea, 1946a).

1.6C

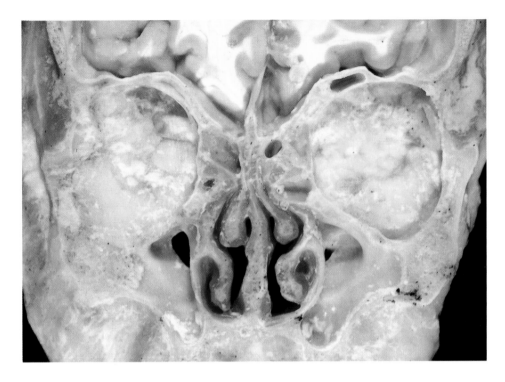

Figure 1.6C. Posterior surface of specimen in Figure 1.6A is shown, which includes the ventral portion of the maxillary sinus.

Figure 1.6D. Residual infundibular and supraorbital cells are shown in this section.

Figure 1.6E. Plain film radiograph of the specimen shown in Figures 1.6A, C.

1.6D

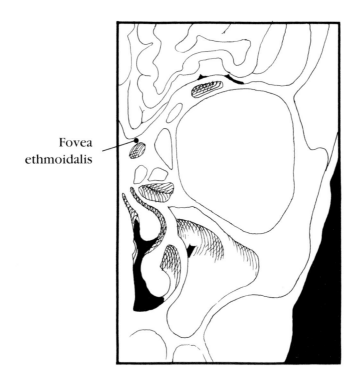

Fovea
ethmoidalis

1.6E

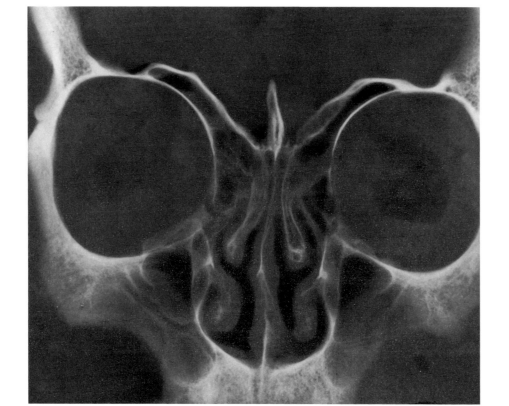

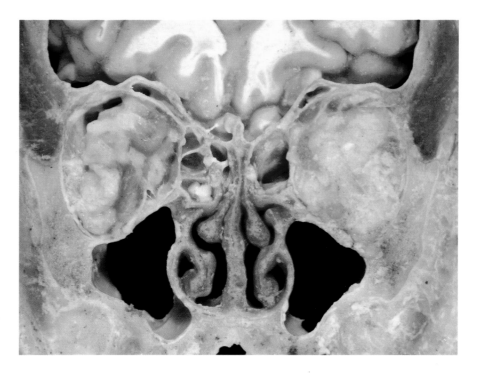

Figure 1.7A. Anterior surface of coronal section contiguous with specimen in Figure 1.6C, is shown, which includes the midportion of the maxillary sinus.

MAXILLARY SINUS

Embryology and Development (Figures 1.1, 1.6, 1.7)

In the third fetal month, an evagination or bud in the infundibulum (also known as the uncibullous groove; Libersa et al., 1981) gives rise to the maxillary sinus. At birth, the sinus has a volume of 6 ml to 8 ml but is fluid-filled, making interpretation of plain film radiography difficult (Schaeffer, 1920; Wasson, 1933). The sinus then undergoes two periods of rapid growth, one between birth and 3 years and the other between 7 and 12 years (Schaeffer, 1910b, 1920). After the second period of rapid growth, subsequent expansion involves pneumatization of the alveolar process of the maxilla. All growth is completed by adulthood, resulting in the descent of the maxillary sinus floor from 4 mm above the floor of the nose at birth to the same level at age 8 to 9 years and, finally, to 4 mm to 5 mm below this site in the adult (Van Alyea, 1951).

Clinical Anatomy

In the adult, the maxillary sinus can be described as triangular, measuring 25 mm along the anterior limb of its base, 34 mm deep, and 33 mm high

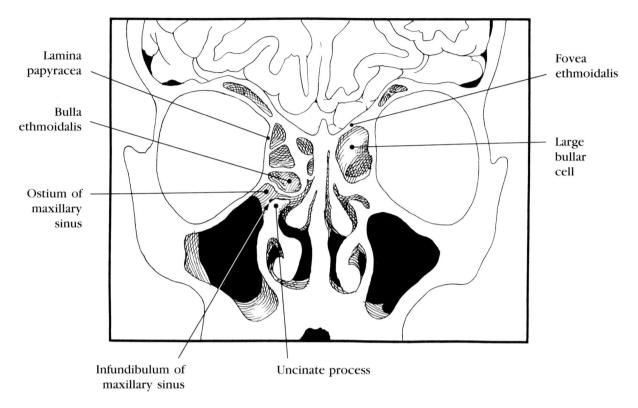

Lamina
papyracea

Bulla
ethmoidalis

Ostium of
maxillary
sinus

Fovea
ethmoidalis

Large
bullar
cell

Infundibulum of
maxillary sinus

Uncinate process

Figure 1.7B. On the right of the specimen are several middle ethmoid cells, including bullar cells. On the left is a large bullar cell.

(Schaeffer, 1920; Van Alyea, 1951). The sinus can be partially compartmentalized by septa, and in rare cases, separate cavities can exist in the posterior part of the sinus, which can be a source of continual infection (Som et al., 1984). The primary ostium, or natural ostium, of this sinus is located in the superior aspect of the medial wall of the sinus and drains into the ethmoid infundibulum or hiatus semilunaris, depending on the terminology (Figure 1.1). Although actual numbers differ with various authors, all agree that most ostia are in the region of the posterior half of the infundibulum or posterior to the midpoint of the bulla ethmoidalis (Schaeffer, 1920; Myerson, 1932; Van Alyea, 1936). The pneumatization of the bulla and the height (e.g., medial and superior projection) of the uncinate process help to form a canal leading to the maxillary sinus, which varies in depth (average 5 mm; Schaeffer, 1910b), orientation, and accessibility via the nose (Myerson, 1932).

The ostium tends to be elliptical, measuring from 1 mm to 20 mm in length (Schaeffer, 1910b). In 15% to 40% of subjects examined by various authors, accessory ostia were found (Schaeffer, 1910b; Van Alyea, 1936; Myerson, 1932). These ostia may be located in the infundibulum or the membranous region of the medial sinus wall, the latter being only a reduplication of the mucosa of the sinus and lateral nasal wall. This region is located inferior to the uncinate process and superior to the insertion of the inferior tur-

1.7C

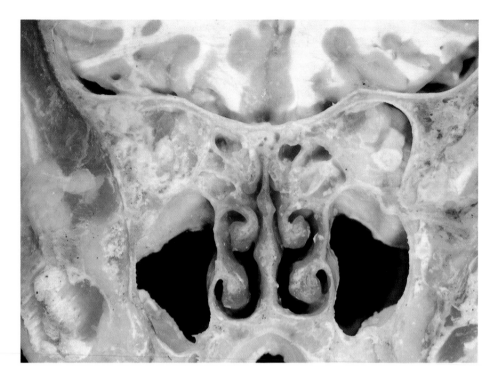

Figure 1.7C. Posterior surface of the specimen in Figure 1.7A is shown, which exposes the middle ethmoid cells.

Figure 1.7D. Illustration showing the middle ethmoid cells seen in Figure 1.7C.

Figure 1.7E. Plain film radiograph of specimen in Figures 1.7A, C. Note the uncinate process projecting several millimeters superiorly (curved arrow). The large arrow points to membranous meatus.

1.7D

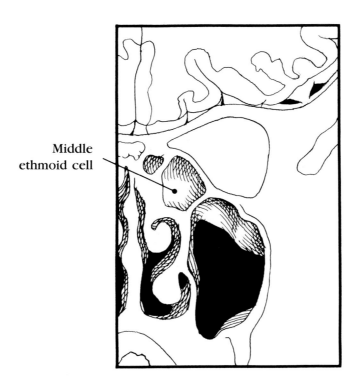

Middle
ethmoid cell

1.7E

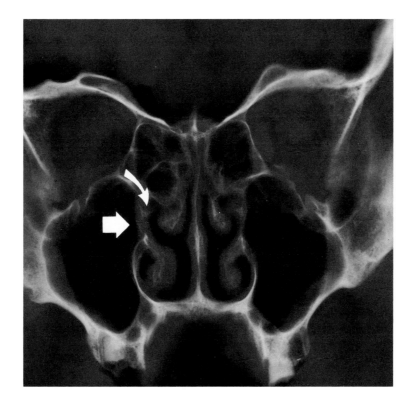

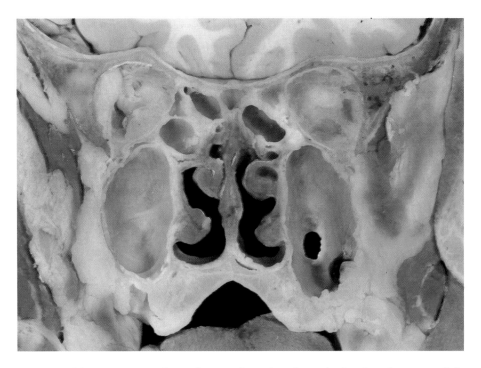

Figure 1.8A. Anterior surface of coronal section through the dorsal aspect of the maxillary sinus is shown.

binate. Clinically, this site is particularly important because it may be used as an alternative to opening the natural ostium when the latter cannot be found during the performance of a supra-inferior turbinate antrostomy.

SPHENOID SINUS

Embryology and Development (Figures 1.1, 1.2, 1.8–1.10)

At birth, the sphenoid sinus is primarily an evagination of the sphenoethmoid recess, with essentially no growth until age 3 years. After this period, the sinus begins to pneumatize the sphenoid bone, and by age 7 years, the sinus extends posteriorly toward the sella turcica. Development may continue into adulthood to involve the basisphenoid, with any possible arrest in development accounting for the tremendous variation in the size of this sinus.

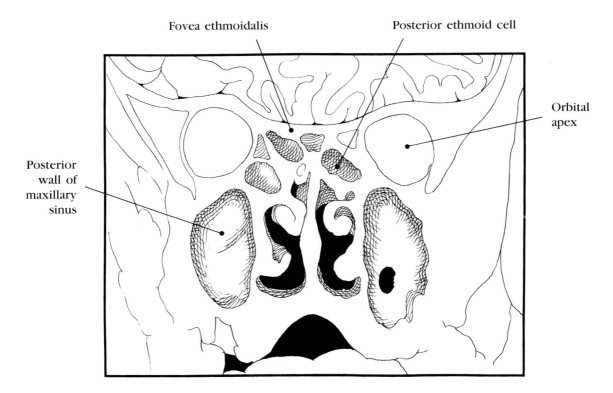

Fovea ethmoidalis   Posterior ethmoid cell

Orbital
apex

Posterior
wall of
maxillary
sinus

Figure 1.8B. Residual maxillary cavity is shown, along with the adjacent posterior ethmoid cells.

Clinical Anatomy

The average adult sinus measures 20 mm high, 23 mm deep, and 17 mm wide (Van Alyea, 1951). The volume varies from 0.1 ml to 30 ml, with the average ranging from 5 ml to 7.5 ml (Dixon, 1937; Van Alyea, 1951). As the sinus expands, vessels and nerves in the lateral aspect of the body of the sphenoid bone come to lie as indentations in the wall of the sinus. Thus, Van Alyea (1951) found a projection of the internal carotid artery into the lateral sinus wall in 65 of 100 heads, with this projection being pronounced in 53 of the specimens (Figure 1.2). In a study of 1,600 skulls, Dixon (1937) found that the optic nerve was present as such an indentation in 8% of the specimens and the vidian nerve in 7%. In this same study, Dixon reported that 22% of the skulls had an intrasinus septum, with dehiscence of the septum observed in only 5 specimens. Equally important is thinning of the superior wall, which may separate the sinus from the dura by only 1 mm (Ritter, 1978).

1.8C

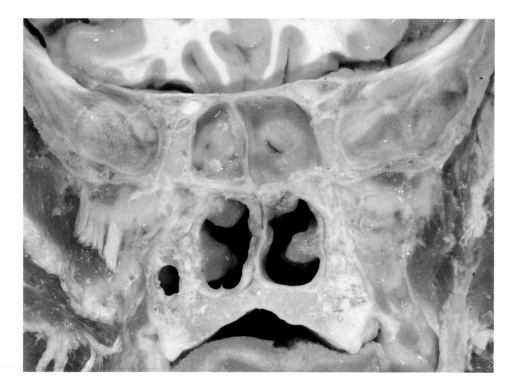

Figure 1.8C. Posterior surface of the specimen in Figure 1.8A is shown. It is immediately dorsal to the maxillary sinus or at the plane of the pterygopalatine space.

Figure 1.8D. Dorsal surface of the anterior wall of the sphenoid sinus is visualized, along with the nasopharynx.

Figure 1.8E. Plain film radiograph of the specimen in Figures 1.8A, C, showing the remnant of the pterygoid plates and the convergence of the posterior ethmoids (Figure 1.8A) and the sphenoid sinus (Figure 1.8C).

1.8D

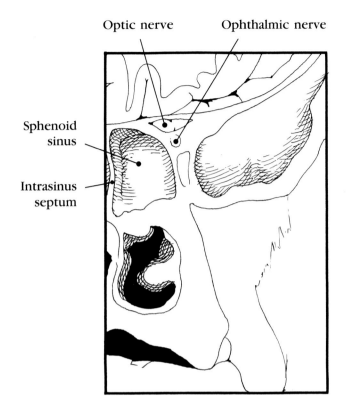

Optic nerve   Ophthalmic nerve

Sphenoid
sinus

Intrasinus
septum

1.8E

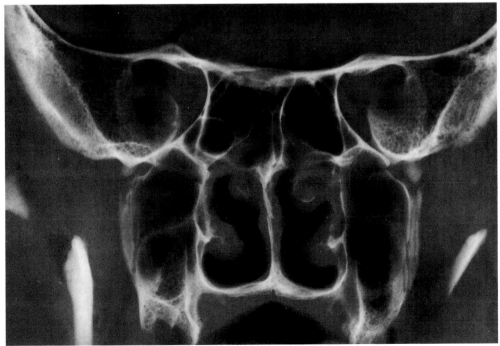
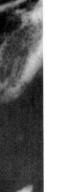

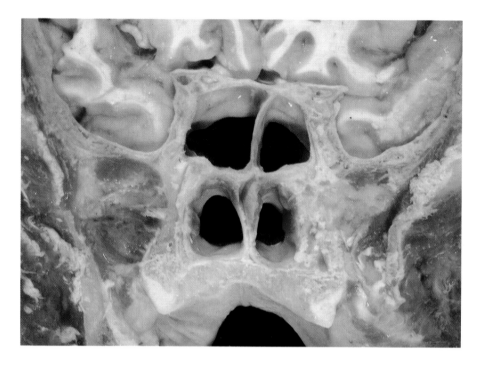

Figure 1.9A. Anterior surface of coronal section contiguous with the specimen in Figure 1.8C, or at a plane adjacent to the dorsal aspect of the anterior wall of the sphenoid sinus.

The sphenoid sinus drains by a single ostium into the sphenoethmoid recess. This ostium, in the clinical setting, is 2 mm to 3 mm in diameter and may be either round or elliptical (Van Alyea, 1951; Dixon, 1937). The sinus depends on mucociliary flow for drainage, since the ostium is located typically 10 mm to 15 mm from the floor of the sinus or 8 mm from the cribriform plate (range 1–15 mm) and 5 mm lateral to the nasal septum, according to Dixon (1937). Our own experience suggests that the ostium tends more often to be inferior than superior to the average location, lying at an angle of 30 degrees from the floor of the nose. In any case, the pneumatization of the posterior aspect of the middle turbinate may make visualization of this ostium difficult. Because of the importance of such identification in surgery, various measurements have been reported (Figure 1.1, Table 1.2).

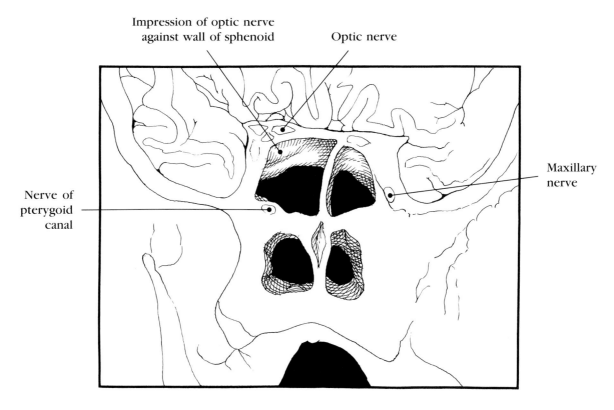

Impression of optic nerve against wall of sphenoid

Optic nerve

Maxillary nerve

Nerve of pterygoid canal

Figure 1.9B. Diagram of Figure 1.9A shows the close proximity of the optic nerve to the sphenoid sinus. Inferior to the sphenoid is the nasopharynx, which appears to be divided into two cavities by the nasal septum.

TABLE 1.2. *Distances in sphenoid sinus*

	Distance from anterior nasal spine	Distance from inferior nasal rim
Sphenoid ostium	7 cm	—
Pituitary fossa	8.5 cm	—
Inferior face of sphenoid	—	5.7 cm
Posterior wall of sphenoid sinus	—	7.6 cm
	Dixon (1937) (in living subjects)	*Mosher (1929)* (in cadavers)

1.9C

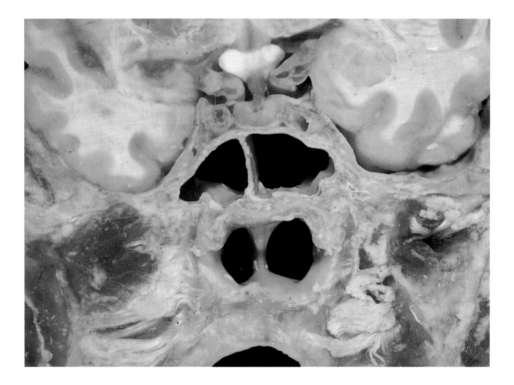

Figure 1.9C. Posterior surface of the specimen in Figure 1.9A, which encompasses the principal cavity of the sphenoid sinus and the pituitary gland.

Figure 1.9D. Note the location of the pituitary gland, internal carotid artery, and optic nerve in relation to the sphenoid sinus.

Figure 1.9E. Plain film radiograph of the specimen in Figures 1.9A, C. The arrow points to the internal carotid artery.

1.9D

Optic
chiasm

Internal carotid
artery

Ophthalmic nerve

Pituitary

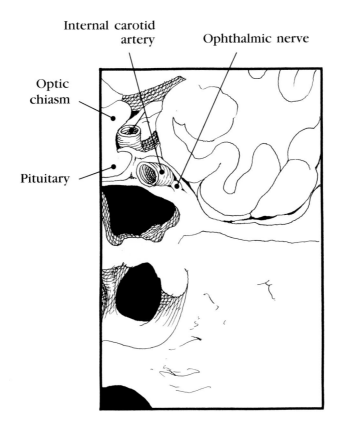

1.9E

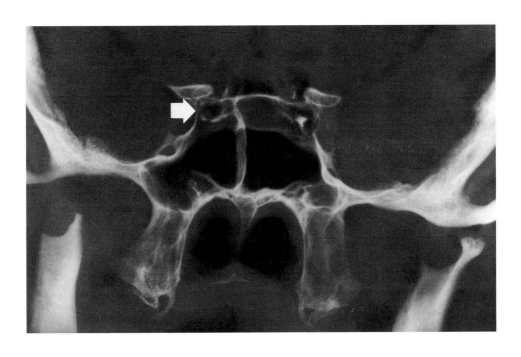

1.10A

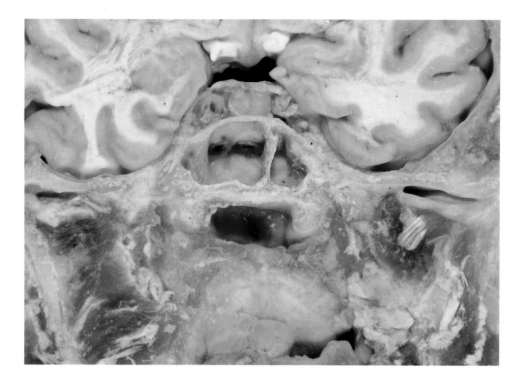

Figure 1.10A. Anterior surface of coronal section contiguous with the section in Figure 1.9C. This is at the plane of the posterior sphenoid sinus.

Figure 1.10B. Drawing of Figure 1.10A. The drawing emphasizes the close relationship of the sphenoid sinus to important neurovascular structures.

Figure 1.10C. Plain film radiograph of specimen in Figure 1.10A. The arrows point to the internal carotid artery.

Internal carotid artery   Pituitary   Right sphenoid sinus   **1.10B**

Impression of
internal carotid
artery against
wall of sphenoid

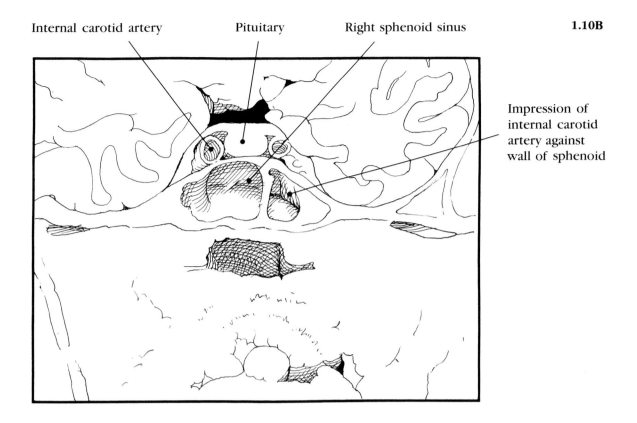

1.10C

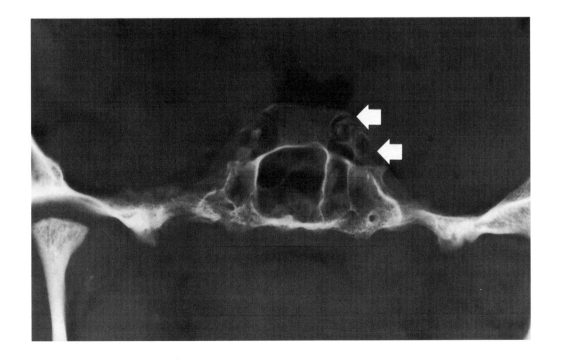

LITERATURE CITED

Blanton, P. L., and Biggs, N. L.
  1969 Eighteen hundred years of controversy: The paranasal sinuses. *Am. J. Anat.,* 124:135–148.

Dixon, F. W.
  1937 A comparative study of the sphenoid. *Ann. Otol. Rhinol. Laryngol.,* 46:687–698.

Hollingshead, W. H.
  1968 *Anatomy for Surgeons: The Head and Neck.* Harper & Row, Hagerstown, MD.

Kasper, K. A.
  1936 Nasofrontal connections. A study based on one hundred consecutive dissections. *Arch. Otolaryngol.,* 23:322–343.

Libersa, C., Laude, M., and Libersa, J.-C.
  1981 The pneumatization of the accessory cavities of the nasal fossae during growth. *Anat. Clin.,* 2:265–278.

Messerklinger, W.
  1985 Endoskopische diagnose und chirurgie der rezidivierenden sinusitis. In: *Advances in Nose and Sinus Surgery,* edited by Z. Krajina. Zagreb University, Zagreb, Yugoslavia.

Mosher, H. P.
  1929 The surgical anatomy of the ethmoidal labyrinth. *Ann. Otol. Rhinol. Laryngol.,* 38:869–901.

Myerson, M. C.
  1932 The natural orifice of the maxillary sinus. I. Anatomic studies. *Arch. Otolaryngol.,* 15:80–91.

Ritter, F. N.
  1978 *The Paranasal Sinuses: Anatomy and Surgical Technique,* 2nd ed. Mosby, St. Louis.

Rosenberger, H. C.
  1938 The clinical availability of the ostium maxillae: A clinical and cadaver study. *Ann. Otol. Rhinol. Laryngol.,* 47:177–182.

Schaeffer, J. P.
  1920 *The Nose, Paranasal Sinuses, Nasolacrimal Passageways, and Olfactory Organ in Man.* Blakiston, Philadelphia.

Schaeffer, J. P.
  1916 The genesis, development, and adult anatomy of the nasofrontal region in man. *Am. J. Anat.,* 20:125–143.

Schaeffer, J. P.
  1912 Types of ostia nasolacrimalia in man and their genetic significance. *Am. J. Anat.,* 13:183–192.

Schaeffer, J. P.
  1910a On the genesis of air cells in the conchae nasales. *Anat. Rec.,* 4:168–180.

Schaeffer, J. P.
  1910b The sinus maxillaris and its relations in the embryo, child, and adult man. *Am. J. Anat.,* 10:313–367.

Shapiro, R., and Janzen, A. H.
  1960 *The Normal Skull: A Roentgen Study.* Paul B. Hoeber, New York.

Simon, E.
  1933 Anatomy of the opening of the maxillary sinus. *Arch. Otolaryngol.,* 29:640–649.

Som, P. M., Sacher, M., Lanzieri, C. F., Lawson, W., and Shuger, J. M.
  1984 The hidden antral compartments. *Radiology,* 152:463–464.

Van Alyea, O. E.
1951 *Nasal Sinuses: An Anatomic and Clinical Consideration,* 2nd ed. Williams & Wilkins, Baltimore.

Van Alyea, O. E.
1946a Frontal sinus drainage. *Ann. Otol. Rhinol. Laryngol.,* 55:267–277.

Van Alyea, O. E.
1946b Maxillary sinus drainage. *Ann. Otol. Rhinol. Laryngol.,* 55:754–763.

Van Alyea, O. E.
1939 Ethmoid labyrinth. Anatomic study, with consideration of the clinical significance of its structural characteristics. *Arch. Otolaryngol.,* 29:881–902.

Van Alyea, O. E.
1941 Frontal cells. An anatomic study of these cells with consideration of their clinical significance. *Arch. Otolaryngol.,* 34:11–23.

Van Alyea, O. E.
1936 The ostium maxillare. Anatomic study of its surgical accessibility. *Arch. Otolaryngol.,* 24:553–569.

Wasson, W. W.
1933 Changes in the nasal accessory sinuses after birth. *Arch. Otolaryngol,* 17:197–211.

Wigand, M. E., Steiner, W., and Jaumann, M. P.
1978 Endonasal sinus surgery with endoscopical control: From radical operation to rehabilitation of the mucosa. *Endoscopy,* 10:255–260.

Wigh, R.
1950 Mucoceles of the fronto-ethmoid sinuses. *Radiology,* 54:579–590.

Zuckerkandl, E.
1893 *Die untere sicbbeinmuschel (mittlere Nasenmuschel), normale und pathologische Anatomie der nasenhohle und ihrer pneumatischen Anhange.* Bd1, Bd2, Wein und Leipzig.

2

Physiology of the Paranasal Sinuses

The sinuses are lined with a ciliated stratified or pseudostratified columnar epithelium. Under this is a tunica propria formed with fibroelastic tissue containing mucous glands and serosanguineous glands. The secretions of these glands combine and form a biphasic mucous blanket that covers the epithelium. This blanket and the ciliated epithelium form the so-called mucociliary system. The mucosa is supplied by both parasympathetic and sympathetic innervation. With stimulation, parasympathetic supply causes an abundant watery flow, and sympathetic stimulation causes a mucinous secretion. The epithelial lining of the sinuses helps supply the nose with a steady covering of mucus to help it warm and humidify the inspired air.

MUCOUS BLANKET

The sinuses are capable of secreting antibacterial and antiviral substances to be carried into the nose. The majority of inspired particulate matter is deposited on the anterior end of the middle and inferior turbinates and in the middle meatus, and the chemicals in the sinus secretions tend to flow toward these areas, thus helping the nose to cleanse the inspired air. Seventy to eighty percent of all particles 3 microns to 5 microns in diameter and

60% of all particles 2 microns in diameter are deposited in the nose (Hilding, 1976). Only particles less than 1 micron in size are able to pass through the nose. The mucous blanket normally contains mast cells, polymorphonuclear leukocytes, eosinophils, lysozyme, and immunoglobulin A, as well as secretory substance (Richmore and Marshall, 1976). It is now the consensus that lysozyme is probably immunoglobulin A plus an immunologic or secretory piece (Tomasi et al., 1965). Immunoglobulin G and interferon also may be found in sinus secretions. The mucous blanket serves also to protect the underlying mucosa.

The upper layer of the mucous blanket is highly viscous, elastic, and tenacious, whereas the lower layer is of lower viscosity, which enables the cilia to move the blanket forward (Lucas and Douglas, 1934). The speed of flow differs in different areas. In the maxillary and frontal sinuses, the direction of flow of the mucus is spiral or circular, centering at the natural ostium. In the sphenoid and ethmoid sinuses, the flow is more or less directly toward the natural ostium. The mucous blanket is renewed in the nose every 10 to 15 minutes (Hilding, 1967). Three types of mucociliary flow have been described: (1) smooth, moving at 0.84 cm per minute, (2) jerky, moving at 0.3 cm per minute, and (3) mucostasis, moving less than 0.3 cm per minute. Both dehydration and low temperature can slow or stop ciliary flow.

The cilia function best in a humid environment. When the relative humidity drops below 50%, ciliary activity is impaired, as it is when the temperature drops below 18°C. Decreased ciliary activity may allow easier penetration and proliferation of bacteria and viruses. Viral diseases cause cellular necrosis, which forms an excellent culture medium for bacteria (Green, 1968). Thus, in acute viral infections, a bacterial component is usually evident within 24 to 48 hours. The mucociliary system attempts to prevent bacterial superinfection. Since most viral upper respiratory infections resolve spontaneously, the system usually is successful. Chronic infection will result only when the system fails. Failure may be caused by a severe infection, by any condition that occludes sinus drainage sufficiently that the mucous blanket is unable to cleanse the sinus, or by ciliary stasis.

SINUS OBSTRUCTION

The maxillary sinus is the first to develop and is present at birth. The natural ostium in the adult is usually 1 mm to 3 mm in size and empties into the middle meatus in the area of the hiatus semilunaris. Accessory ostia are frequent. Partial or complete block of the natural ostium is usual in either acute or chronic disease. The ethmoid cells from the beginning are divided into two primary groups by the attached lateral border and lamina of the middle turbinate. The anterior ethmoid cells empty into the infundibulum along with the frontal sinus. Secretions from here drain across the maxillary ostium. Thus, obstruction in the area of the hiatus semilunaris may obstruct these three sinuses.

Chronic or chronic–recurrent sinusitis, therefore, implies a breakdown in the mucociliary system. This breakdown usually involves the anterior ethmoids, which are ideally located and anatomically constructed to suffer chronic obstruction; the numerous small air cells with their narrow ostia are obstructed easily. Chronic infection here will produce edema of the surrounding mucosa. Experience examining and operating on these patients demonstrates the ease with which such mucosal edema can obstruct the maxillary and frontal sinuses. Numerous insults may cause obstruction here, the most common being acute viral or bacterial infections and acute allergic reactions. The posterior ethmoid sinuses may drain through the anterior ethmoid sinuses or posteriorly. The sphenoid sinus drains independently, but its ostium may be obstructed by edema involving the posterior ethmoid sinuses or the posterior end of the middle turbinate.

Chronic Sinusitis and Infections

Bronchopulmonary infections frequently may be associated with chronic sinusitis, particularly in children, and treating one condition is usually unsuccessful without treating the other. Sasaki and Kirschner (1967) pointed out three possible routes of infection in the sinobronchial syndrome: (1) tracheal aspiration, (2) lymphatic–hematogenous route, and (3) purely lymphatic pathway. Regardless of the pathway, an interrelationship between hyperplastic sinusitis and chronic bronchopulmonary infections seems clear from the available evidence. Problems have resulted from the overenthusiastic use of a single treatment modality, such as surgery alone or medication alone, directed at only one problem.

NASAL AIRWAY

The nose is the most important respiratory organ, since ororespiration is unphysiologic and acquired. Oral respiration should be used only in short periods of increased ventilatory demands. Nasal breathing allows more time for maximum gas diffusion in the pulmonary alveoli because it is slower and deeper than oral breathing (Arnott et al., 1968). The nose acts as a variable resistor and accounts for as much as 40% of total airway resistance. During normal respiration, pressure changes in the nasal cavity approximate 6 cm of water, and flow rates average 15 liters per minute (Hilding, 1976).

One factor that affects the diameter of the nasal vault is the nasal cycle. This, in addition to the autonomic nervous system, which can change the mucosal thickness in situations of anxiety or pain, controls nasal airway resistance. It is well known that, in the normal nose, one nasal airway opens, with increased secretion from serous and mucous glands, while the opposite airway closes, with nearly complete cessation of secretion. The open and closed sides switch every 2 to 3 hours. The explanation for this is unknown, but it may be the reason for a nasal septum. Sleeping position affects the filling of the erectile tissue of the nasal cavity, and the turbinates on the dependent side reach their maximum size in 15 to 20 minutes. When one turns, the up side of the nose opens and the down side congests in 10 to 15 minutes (Heetderks, 1927). This nasal cycle is present in about 80% of normal people. Kerning (1968) studied 17 young adults with normal noses on rhinoscopy and found regular cycles in 7 that were individually characteristic, ranging from 2 to 7 hours. In 6 others there were no patency reversals, and in 4 there were irregular cycles. The factor that controls the cycle is unknown, but the cycle continues despite anesthetizing of the nasal mucosa.

Sinus ostium patency depends on the size of the bony aperture and on the thickness of the mucosa. Even a small change in the thickness of the mucosa can produce profound effects, since the area of the opening is reduced as the square of the radius. Thus, any kind of nasal vasomotor response, either normal, as in the nasal cycle, allergic, or inflammatory, can obstruct the sinus ostium. The functional integrity of the sinuses is dependent to a large measure on nasal breathing. This is illustrated by the fact that oxygen exchange between the nose and the sinuses is twice as high in nasal breathing as it is in mouth breathing and is inversely proportional to nasal air flow and nasal breathing pressure. In the normal nasal cycle, this relative obstruction, decrease in amount of secretion, and decrease in oxygen exchange do not persist long enough for infection to occur. Something else must occur to block the sinus or impair the mucociliary system for a longer period for infection to occur.

SINUS FUNCTION

The function of the sinuses is unknown. It has been stated that one of the functions is to impart a resonance to the voice, but many studies on voice resonance in humans have failed to find a convincing relationship. Another function that has been stated is to warm and humidify inspired air, but clearly, the air exchange between the nose and sinuses makes this function insignificant when compared to this function in the nose. Regarding the function of regulating intranasal pressure, Suarez (1952) found that when the sinuses are occluded by disease, variations in nasal pressure are not quite as great as they are otherwise. He concluded that the function of the sinuses is to keep the pressure in the nose within certain boundaries and to dampen the high pressures that accompany such acts as sneezing and nose blowing. However, the small average volume of the sinuses, which is approximately 45 ml, is too minute to mitigate the high pressures developed during sneezing. Sinuses do form some sort of shock absorber, but the effectiveness is variable depending on pneumatization of the sinuses.

The sinuses secrete some mucus to help the nasal cavity, but this seems to be a small amount compared to the total volume secreted. However, the location of the ostia of the frontal, maxillary, and anterior ethmoid sinuses is such as to supply what mucus it does where it is needed most. This is in the middle meatus, where it would be most effective in helping cleanse the nose of particulate matter deposited during normal nasal respiration.

The key points relative to endoscopic sinus surgery are the mucociliary system and the location of the ostia. The integrity of this mucociliary system must be maintained to prevent bacterial infection of the sinuses. The anterior ethmoid sinuses are located at a point where they and the frontal and maxillary sinuses drain. Any event that occludes the anterior ethmoid sinuses could lead to mucosal inflammation sufficient to occlude the other sinuses. The object of endoscopic sinus surgery is to create a situation anatomically that will obviate obstruction and ostial occlusion in this area.

LITERATURE CITED

Arbour, P., and Kern, E. B.
  1975 Paradoxical nasal obstruction. *Can. J. Otolaryngol.,* 4:333–338.
Arnott, W. M., Cumming, G., and Horsfield, K.
  1968 Alveolar ventilation. *Ann. Intern. Med.,* 69:1–12.
Green, R. N.
  1968 The role of viral infection in the etiology and pathogenesis of chronic bronchitis and emphysema, with consideration of a naturally occurring animal model. *Yale J. Biol. Med.,* 40:461–476.
Grossman, M.
  1975 The saccharin test of nasal mucociliary function. *Eye Ear Nose Throat,* 54:415.
Heetderks, D. L.
  1927 Observations on the reactions of normal nasal mucous membrane. *Am. J. Med. Sci.,* 174:231.
Hilding, A. C.
  1976 Nasal filtration. In: Hinchcliffe R, Harrison D. *Scientific Foundations of Otolaryngology,* edited by R. Hinchcliffe and D. Harrison, pp. 502–512. Year Book, Chicago.
Hilding, A. C.
  1967 The role of the respiratory mucosa in health and disease. *Minn. Med.,* 50:915–919.
Kerning, J.
  1968 On the nasal cycle. *Rhinol. Int.,* 6:99–136.
Lucas, A. M., and Douglas, L. C.
  1934 Principles underlying ciliary activity in the respiratory tract. II. A comparison of nasal clearance in man, monkey and other mammals. *Arch. Otolaryngol.,* 20:518–541.
Richmore, J. T., and Marshall, M. L.
  1976 Cytology of nasal secretions: Further diagnostic help. *Laryngoscope,* 86:516.
Sasaki, C. T., and Kirchner, J. A.
  1967 A lymphatic pathway from the sinuses to the mediastinum. *Arch. Otolaryngol.,* 85:432–444.
Suarez, A.
  1952 Una nueva teoria sobre la function de los senos paranasales y celdas-daas. *Rev. Egs. Otoneurooftalmol. Neurocir.,* 11:336.
Tomasi, T. B., Tan, E. M., Soloman, A., and Pendergast, R. A.
  1965 Characteristics of immune system common to certain external secretions. *J. Exp. Med.,* 121:101–124.

Radiology of the Paranasal Sinuses

Terry S. Becker and Barbara Zeifer Ukra

Functional endoscopic sinus surgery (ESS) is based on the premise that primary inflammatory disease in the middle meatus, anterior ethmoid, and maxillary sinus ostium (ostiomeatal unit, or OMU) causes secondary sinusitis, particularly in the maxillary and frontal sinuses. Although the symptomatology related to these secondary findings may predominate, it is the primary disease in the OMU that must be eradicated for clinical improvement to occur.

Messerklinger (1967, 1978), studying mucociliary drainage of the paranasal sinuses, showed that apposition of mucosal surfaces causes ventilatory disturbance in the OMU. Whether caused by infection or anatomic malformation, the result is decreased mucociliary clearance of the frontal and maxillary sinuses, resulting in recurrent sinusitis. Although Hilding (1944) had shown in cadaver material that mucociliary clearance in the maxillary sinus drains to the natural ostium, circumventing surgical openings such as nasoantral windows, the significance of this finding was not recognized. Intranasal antrostomy and the Caldwell-Luc procedure remained mainstays in the surgical management of chronic recurrent sinusitis.

It is now recognized that subtle mucosal change in the OMU is the substrate for chronic sinusitis. This, combined with the advent of more sophisticated endoscopic equipment, has enabled the head and neck surgeon to provide a truly physiologic operation to the patient with chronic recurrent

Figure 3.1. Use of off-coronal scan.

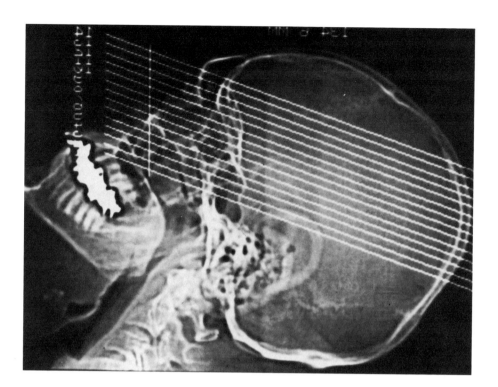

Figure 3.1A. Scout view examination. Gantry is tilted as shown by cursor lines to avoid dental amalgams.

sinusitis. Stammberger (1986) has shown that varying degrees of inflammatory disease in the OMU can be eradicated successfully by this technique. Kennedy et al. (1985) have clarified and popularized ESS in the United States.

Computed tomography (CT) plays a critical role in the preoperative evaluation of patients considered for ESS. CT is sensitive in identifying minor inflammatory or anatomic changes in the OMU that are responsible for the secondary changes of chronic frontal and maxillary sinusitis (Zinreich et al., 1987). Plain film radiography is relatively insensitive in the evaluation of these subtle changes. Pluridirectional tomography, although more reliable than plain films, is inferior to CT and produces higher radiation exposure.

Systematic nasal endoscopy acts as a complement to CT, providing excellent visualization of the middle meatus. Endoscopy, however, may not provide visualization of the ethmoid infundibulum or maxillary sinus ostium. Furthermore, CT is able to identify deep mucosal changes that cannot be visualized by endoscopy. CT can identify anatomic abnormalities or variants that are important in preoperative evaluation. CT, therefore, is important in preoperative planning and plays a significant role in patient selection.

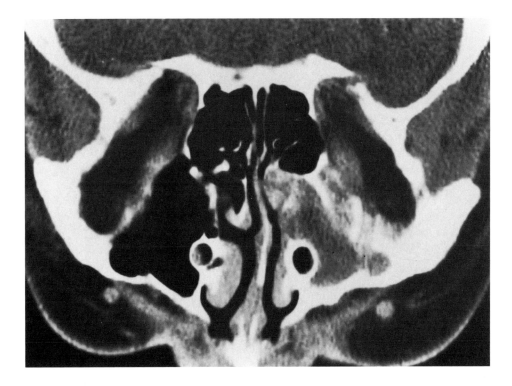

Figures 3.1B. Scan obtained 45 degrees off the coronal plane adequately demonstrates the relationship between the maxillary sinus, middle meatus, and ethmoid sinus.

COMPUTED TOMOGRAPHY TECHNIQUE

Relatively thin section thickness (5 mm) contiguous scans are obtained in the direct coronal plane. Patients may be scanned in either the supine or the prone position. In patients who cannot tolerate direct coronal positioning or in whom dental amalgams may cause artifacts, axial scans with coronal reformations may be helpful (Zinreich et al., 1987). Reformatted views, in our experience, however, are inferior to direct coronal images and are not a part of our practice. Instead, where coronal scans are not obtainable or are limited by dental amalgam artifact, we image the patient in the off-coronal plane, easily obtained with patient positioning or gantry angulation (Figure 3.1A, B).

Examinations are performed without intravenous contrast. The image size should be targeted to allow the paranasal sinuses to fill the screen or film frame. Soft tissue windows (window width/level of 350/50) are obtained. In addition, low window setting levels similar to those used for lung CT imaging (window width/level of 2,000/−500) are obtained for enhancement of mucosal detail (Figure 3.2A, B). These numerical values are approximate and should be adjusted for each scanner–camera combination. Bone windows (windows width/level of 1,500/400) are occasionally useful when marked mucosal thickening or soft tissue masses are present but are not obtained routinely.

Figure 3.2. Use of CT windows setting.

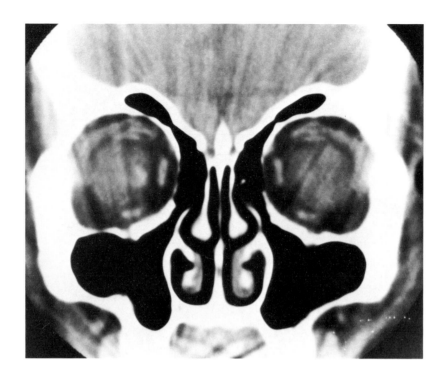

Figure 3.2A. Conventional soft tissue windows (CT window width/level 350/50).

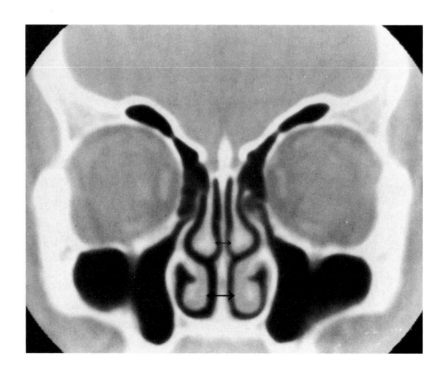

Figure 3.2B. By using a wide CT window width and low level (2,000/−500), mucosal and soft tissue contrast is exaggerated. Note the normal mucosa of the turbinates (arrows) as well as a septum in the right maxillary sinus not identified in Figure 3.2A.

NORMAL CORONAL COMPUTED TOMOGRAPHY ANATOMY OF PARANASAL SINUSES

The anatomy of the soft tissues, bony margins, and air-containing spaces is well visualized by CT (Hesselink et al., 1978; Schatz and Becker, 1984). As noted previously, the coronal plane is preferred, most accurately demonstrating the air spaces and OMU. The most anterior coronal section (Figure 3.3A) includes the frontal sinus and anterior nasal fossae. Slightly posterior, at the level of the anterior ethmoid and maxillary sinuses (Figure 3.3B), the middle and inferior turbinate may be visualized. The nasolacrimal canal containing the lacrimal duct is visualized in this plane and should not be mistaken for the ethmoid infundibulum or middle meatus.

More posteriorly, the maxillary sinus communicates with the middle meatus and anterior ethmoid sinus (Figure 3.3C). The maxillary sinus ostium opens into the hiatus semilunaris through a slitlike opening, the ethmoid infundibulum. The infundibulum is bordered medially by the uncinate process and superiolaterally by the ethmoid bulla and orbital floor.

Identification of the middle meatus–anterior ethmoid–maxillary sinus ostium complex (OMU) in the coronal plane is important for the evaluation of subtle mucosal thickening that predisposes to secondary inflammatory change in the maxillary sinus.

The posterior ethmoid sinus (Figure 3.3D) is separated from the maxillary sinus by the ethmoidomaxillary plate, from the orbit by the posterior aspect of the lamina papyracea, and from the anterior cranial fossa by the planum sphenoidale. The sphenoid sinus (Figure 3.3E) is separated from the posterior ethmoid by the sphenoethmoidal recess, not usually identified on coronal scans. Sphenoid sinus pneumatization, its asymmetrical septum, and relationship to the posterior choanae, nasopharynx, and surrounding bony margins are well visualized.

Anatomic variants in the paranasal sinuses and nasal fossa may be recognized on CT. These variants occasionally may predispose to or exaggerate inflammatory changes. Their identification also is important in operative planning. Marked enlargement of the ethmoid bulla, lateral rotation of the uncinate process, and lateral convexity of the middle turbinate may cause ventilatory disturbances. A concha bullosa (Figure 3.4) represents pneumatization of the middle turbinate. When large, the concha bullosa may narrow the middle meatus. Similarly, a deviated septum (Figure 3.4) may result in middle meatus narrowing and impaired ventilation of the OMU.

TABLE 3.1. *Key to illustrations*

1. Frontal sinus	9. Middle turbinate	17. Lamina papyracea
2. Cartilagenous nasal septum	10. Inferior turbinate	18. Planum sphenoidale
3. Vomer	11. Maxillary sinus ostium	19. Sphenoid sinus
4. Perpendicular plate of the ethmoid	12. Ethmoid infundibulum	20. Pterygoid plates
5. Anterior ethmoid sinus	13. Uncinate process of the ethmoid	21. Sphenoidal keel (rostrum)
6. Maxillary sinus	14. Ethmoid bulla	22. Superior orbital fissure
7. Nasolacrimal canal	15. Posterior ethmoid sinus	23. Foramen rotundum
8. Middle meatus	16. Ethmoidomaxillary plate	24. Anterior clinoid process

Figure 3.3. Normal Coronal CT Anatomy of the Paranasal Sinuses.

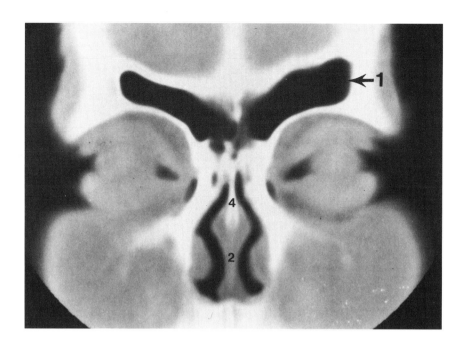

Figure 3.3A. The most anterior section demonstrates the frontal sinus (1) arising above the nasal fossa, which is divided by the cartilagenous nasal septum (2), vomer, and perpendicular plate of the ethmoid (4).

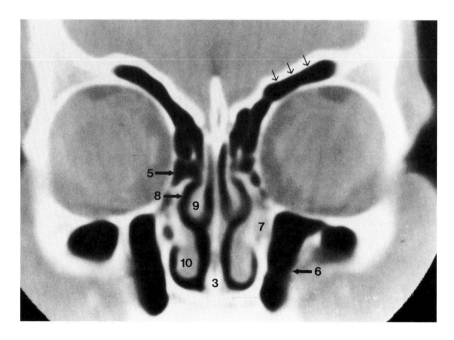

Figure 3.3B. Section 5 mm posterior to that in Figure 3.3A. The anterior aspect of the ethmoid (5) and maxillary sinus (6) is visible. Supra-orbital ethmoid air cell extension is present (arrows). The left nasolacrimal canal (7) courses medial to the maxillary sinus and should not be confused with the middle meatus or the ethmoid infundibulum, which are more posterior. The middle meatus (8) and turbinate (9), inferior meatus and turbinate (10), and vomer (3) are well visualized.

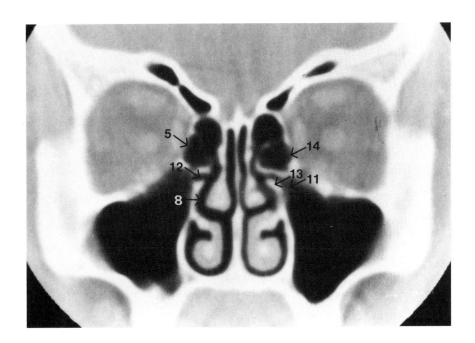

Figure 3.3C. The ostiomeatal unit is formed by the anterior ethmoid (5), middle meatus (8), and maxillary sinus ostium (11). It includes the ethmoid infundibulum (12) bordered by the uncinate process of the ethmoid medially (13) and the ethmoid bulla (14) and floor of the orbit superolaterally.

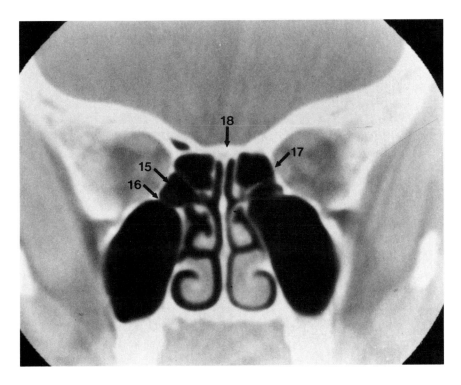

Figure 3.3D. The posterior ethmoid sinus (15) is separated from the maxillary sinus by the ethmoidomaxillary plate (16), from the orbit by the lamina papyracea (17), and from the anterior cranial fossa by the planum sphenoidale (18).

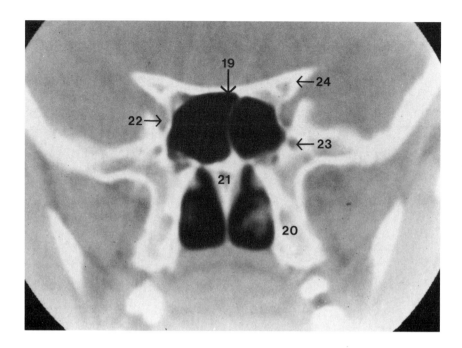

Figure 3.3E. The sphenoid sinus (19) is well aerated. The septum as shown here is usually asymmetrical. Also visualized are the pterygoid plates (20), sphenoidal keel (21), superior orbital fissure (22), foramen rotundum (23), and anterior clinoid process (24).

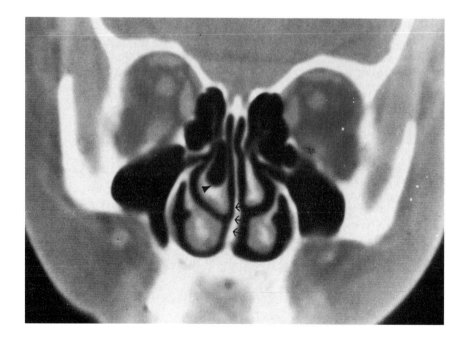

Figure 3.4. Anatomic variants. Although no inflammatory mucosal changes are present, there is noted a large concha bullosa (pneumatized middle turbinate; arrowhead), resulting in a slightly narrowed middle meatus. Mild leftward nasal septal deviation is present (arrows).

PATHOLOGIC ANATOMY

As noted previously, coronal CT imaging of the OMU is critical before ESS. Subtle areas of mucosal thickening are well demonstrated in the region of the maxillary sinus ostium, ethmoid infundibulum, and middle meatus. In addition, secondary mucosal thickening of the lateral and inferior maxillary sinus, as well as frontal and sphenoid sinusitis, may be visualized.

In severe cases (Figure 3.5A), extensive mucosal masses obliterating the OMU are evident. Secondary mucosal thickening in the frontal or sphenoid sinus is observed (Figure 3.5B). Soft tissue thickening in the middle meatus is most frequent (Zinreich et al., 1987). In more moderate cases of inflammatory disease, subtle soft tissue thickening (Figure 3.6) in the ethmoid infundibulum and middle meatus must be sought.

Mucosal thickening is usually bilateral, although asymmetry is the rule. In the presence of incomplete or intermittent ostium and infundibular occlusion, the ostium may appear clear in the presence of ethmoid or maxillary sinus inflammatory change (Figures 3.7A, B, 3.8). In case where CT findings are atypical or minimal, the decision to perform ESS or to continue medical therapy is more difficult.

Figure 3.5. Severe bilateral ostiomeatal disease.

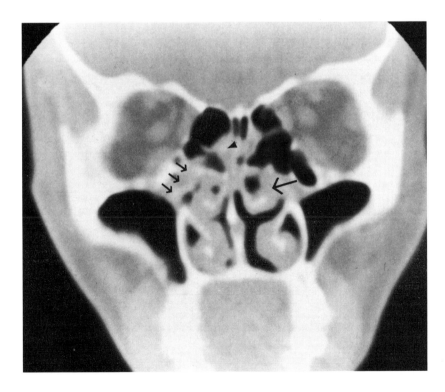

Figure 3.5A. Anteriorly, marked mucosal thickening involves the ostia of the maxillary sinuses and ethmoid infundibula (small arrows). Marked mucosal soft tissue density is present in the anterior ethmoid (arrowhead) and middle meatus (large arrow).

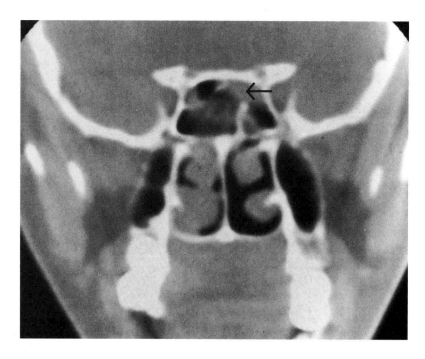

Figure 3.5B. Associated sphenoid sinusitis is noted posteriorly (arrow).

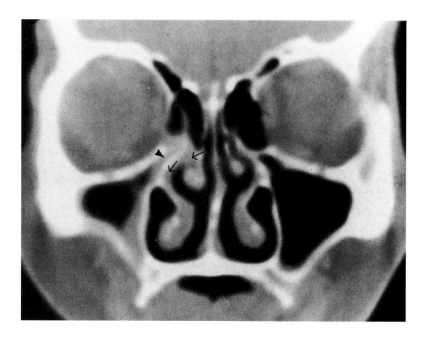

Figure 3.6. Moderate right ostiomeatal disease. Mucosal thickening obliterates the ethmoid infundibulum (arrowhead), extending to the anterior ethmoid sinus. Slight mucosal thickening is present in the middle meatus (arrows). Associated mild mucosal thickening is present in the right maxillary sinus medially.

Figure 3.7. Bilateral ostiomeatal disease.

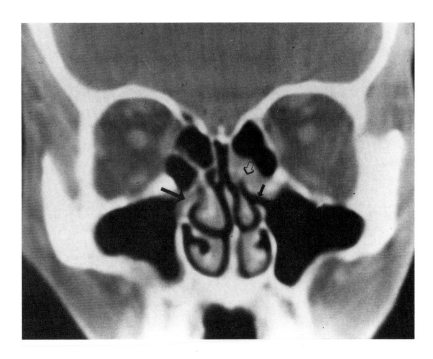

Figure 3.7A. The right maxillary sinus ostium and ethmoid infundibulum are obliterated by inflamed mucosa (large arrow). Although the left maxillary sinus ostium and ethmoid infundibulum are clear (small arrow), moderate left ethmoid mucosal thickening is present (open arrow).

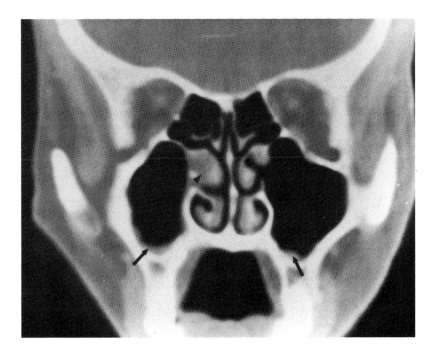

Figure 3.7B. More posteriorly marked mucosal thickening of the right middle meatus is present (arrowhead). Minimal mucosal thickening is present in the floor of the maxillary sinuses bilaterally (arrows).

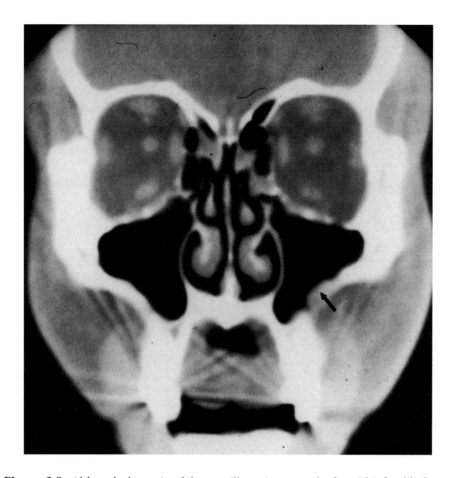

Figure 3.8. Although the ostia of the maxillary sinuses and ethmoid infundibula are clear, mild mucosal thickening is present in the anterior ethmoid sinuses. Slight mucosal thickening is present in the floor of the left maxillary sinus (arrow).

POSTOPERATIVE COMPUTED TOMOGRAPHY

CT is not recommended routinely after ESS, since clinical improvement is the keystone in evaluating surgical success. CT, however, will show clearing of the ostiomeatal disease and varying degrees of improvement within the rest of the sinuses (Figures 3.9A, B, 3.10A, B). In patients with persistent symptomatology after conventional surgery or in patients who have not improved adequately within 4 to 8 months after ESS, CT may be of value, demonstrating persistent mucosal inflammatory changes superimposed on variable surgical defects (Figure 3.11A, B).

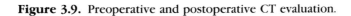

Figure 3.9. Preoperative and postoperative CT evaluation.

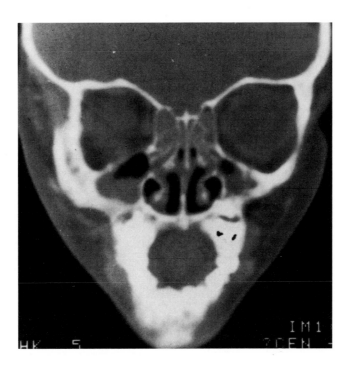

Figure 3.9A. Preoperative CT. Marked bilateral ostiomeatal disease with associated maxillary and ethmoid sinusitis.

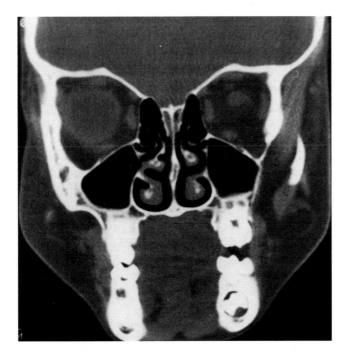

Figure 3.9B. CT 10 weeks postoperatively. Except for minimal residual mucosal thickening in the floor of the left maxillary sinus, complete clearing has occurred.

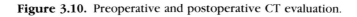

Figure 3.10. Preoperative and postoperative CT evaluation.

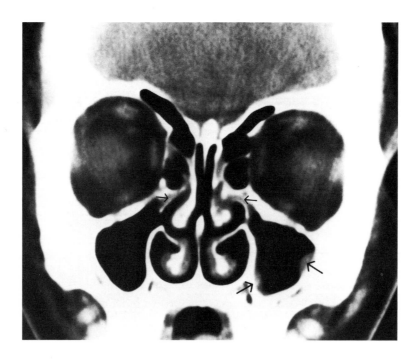

Figure 3.10A. Preoperative CT. Minimal mucosal thickening of both ostiomeatal units and inferior left maxillary sinus (arrows).

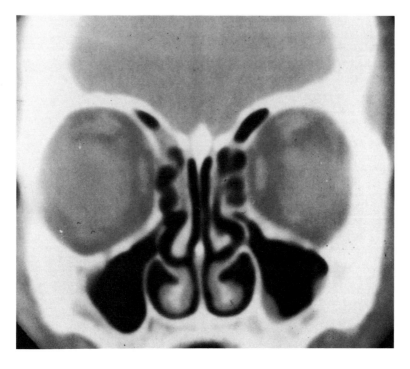

Figure 3.10B. Nine months postoperative CT. Ostia of the maxillary sinuses and ethmoid infundibula are clear, although minimal mucosal thickening of the ethmoids and left maxillary sinus persists. Patient was asymptomatic.

Figure 3.11. Postoperative CT evaluation. Twenty-two-year-old man with persistent symptoms after right ethmoidectomy, polypectomy, and nasoantral window.

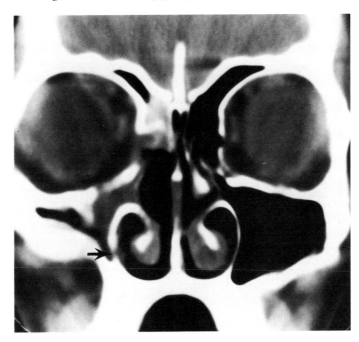

Figure 3.11A. Marked mucosal thickening is evident in the left ethmoid infundibulum and maxillary and ethmoid sinuses. Small right nasoantral window is present (arrow).

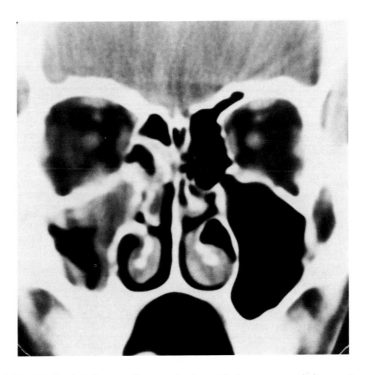

Figure 3.11B. Marked right maxillary and ethmoid sinus mucosal disease is evident posteriorly.

LITERATURE CITED

Hesselink, J. R., New, P. F. J., Davis, K. R., et al.
  1978 Computed tomography of the paranasal sinuses and face. Part I. Normal anatomy. *J. Comput. Assist. Tomogr.*, 2:559–567.

Hilding, A. C.
  1944 The physiology of nasal mucus. IV. Drainage of the accessory sinuses in man. *Ann. Otol. Rhinol. Laryngol.*, 53:35–41.

Kennedy, D. W., Zinreich, S. J., Rosenbaum, A. E., and Johns, M. E.
  1985 Functional endoscopic sinus surgery, theory and diagnostic evaluation. *Arch. Otolaryngol.*, 111:576–582.

Messerklinger, W.
  1978 *Endoscopy of the Nose.* Urban and Schwartzenberg, Baltimore.

Messerklinger, W.
  1967 On the drainage of the normal frontal sinus of man. *Acta Otolaryngol.*, 63:176–181.

Schatz, C. J., and Becker, T. S.
  1984 Normal CT anatomy of the paranasal sinuses. *Radiol. Clin. North Am.*, 22:107–118.

Stammberger, H.
  1986 Endoscopic endonasal surgery—Concepts in treatment of recurring rhinosinusitis. Part 1. Anatomic and pathophysiologic considerations. *Otolaryngol. Head Neck Surg.*, 94:143–155.

Zinreich, S. J., Kennedy D. W., Rosenbaum, A. E., et al.
  1987 Paranasal sinuses: CT imaging requirements for endoscopic surgery. *Radiology*, 163:769–775.

4

Patient and Equipment Selection

OFFICE ENDOSCOPY

Office endoscopy forms the cornerstone of building a competent foundation for managing the patient with paranasal sinus disease in the office and operating room. The novice sinus endoscopist's first step should be to gain familiarity with and then expertise in office examination of the nose with optical telescopes.

Routine Examination of the Nose

The physician should develop a standard method for evaluating patients with sinus disease. Since such disease frequently is caused by obstruction of the ostia of the sinuses, each of these sites, along with the nasal septum, must be visualized. To accomplish this, one must first have at least one standard 30-degree (and possibly one standard 70-degree) telescope or one wide-angle 25- or 30-degree telescope, a light cord, and a light source in the office. Such telescopes are available in 4.0 and 2.7 mm diameters (Figure 4.1). The larger telescopes offer a slightly better view of the nose, whereas the smaller ones are easier to use, particularly in children.

Figure 4.1. Representative endoscopic sinus surgery instruments currently manufactured. For additional equipment available, refer to manufacturers' catalogues.

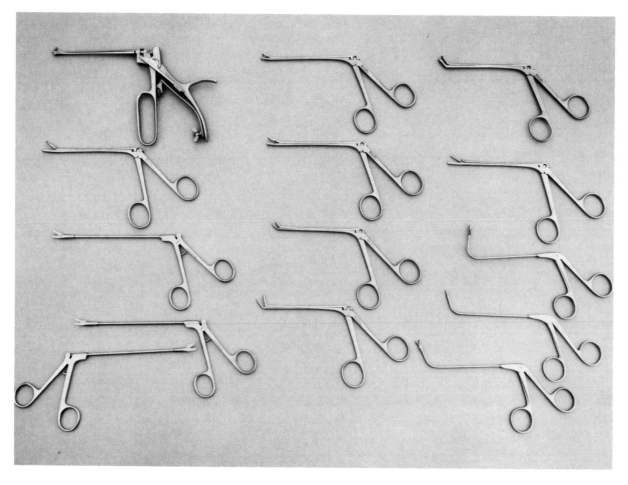

Figure 4.1A. Richards Medical Company endoscopic sinus surgery instruments.

Retrograde forceps on universal handle	Weil-Blakesley forceps (straight, size 1)	Weil-Blakesley forceps (upturned, size 3)
Weil-Blakesley forceps (straight, size 3)	Weil-Blakesley forceps (straight, size 2)	Struychen nasal cutter
Turbinate scissors (straight)	Weil-Blakesley forceps (upturned, size 1)	Double spoon forceps (100-degree angle, horizontal cutting)
Turbinate scissors (left)	90-degree Weil-Blakesley forceps (size 3)	Punch biopsy forceps (70-degree angle)
Turbinate scissors (right)		Double spoon forceps (70-degree angle, vertical cutting)

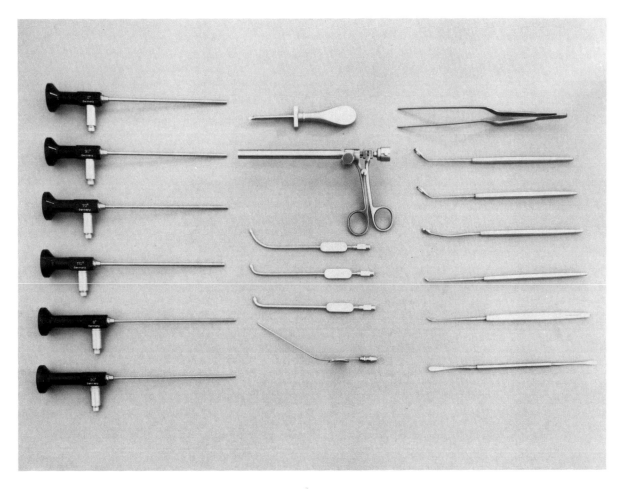

Figure 4.1B. Richards Medical Company endoscopic sinus surgery instruments (continued).

0-degree Wide angle 4.0 mm telescope	5 mm Trocar and cannula	Packing forceps
30-degree Wide-angle 4.0 mm telescope	Optical forceps	Antral curette (forward cutting)
70-degree Wide-angle 4.0 mm telescope	4 mm Bent suction	Antral curette (backward cutting)
110-degree Wide-angle 4.0 mm telescope	Antrum cannula (small)	Antral curette (oval)
0-degree 2.7 mm Telescope	Antrum cannula (large)	Antral curette (oblong)
30-degree 2.7 mm Telescope	No. 5 suction	Sickle knife (pointed)
		Freer elevator

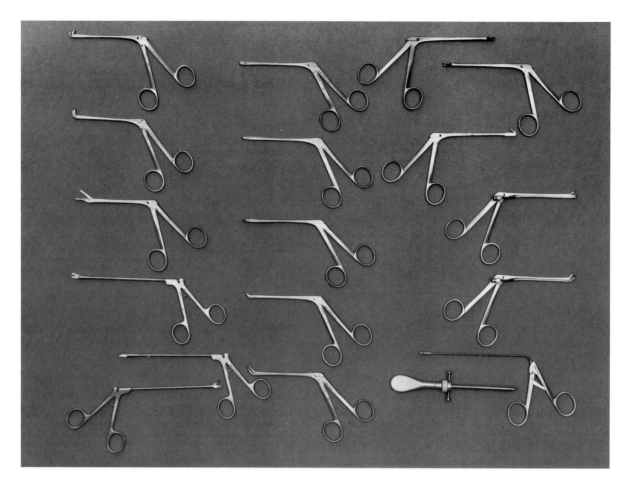

Figure 4.1C. Karl Storz Endoscopy–America endoscopic sinus surgery instruments.

90-degree Blakesley-Wilde forceps (size 1)	Takahashi forceps (size 1)	Stammberger antrum punch (sideward cutting, right)
90-degree Blakesley-Wilde forceps (size 2)	Blakesley forceps (size 1)	Stammberger antral punch (sideward cutting, left)
Struycken nasal cutter	Blakesley forceps (size 4)	Stammberger antral punch (backward cutting)
Nasal scissors (straight)	Strumpel-Voss forceps (upturned)	Blakesley suction punch (straight, size 1)
Nasal scissors (left)	Blakesley-Wilde forceps (upturned, size 2)	Blakesley suction punch (curved, size 1)
Nasal scissors (right)		Biopsy forceps
		5 mm Trocar and cannula (oblique beak)

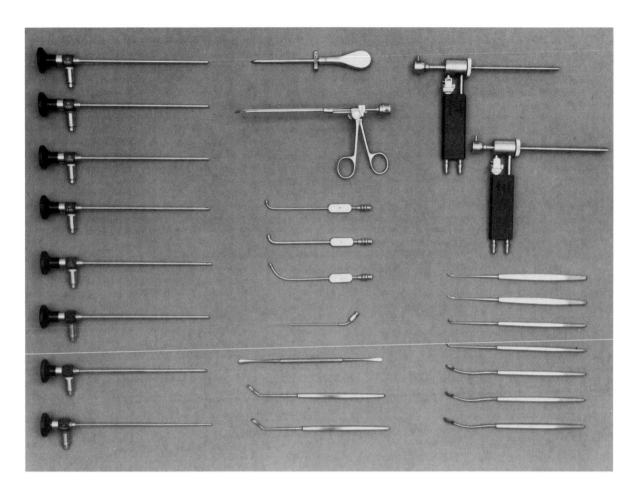

Figure 4.1D. Karl Storz Endoscopy–America endoscopic sinus surgery instruments (continued).

0-degree 4 mm Telescope	5 mm Trocar and cannula	Suction and irrigation sheath with handle for 30-degree telescope
30-degree 4 mm Telescope	Optical forceps	Suction and irrigation sheath with handle for 70-degree telescope
70-degree 4 mm Telescope	Antrum cannula (size 1)	Sickle knife (blunt)
90-degree 4 mm Telescope	Antrum cannula (size 2)	Sickle knife (pointed)
120-degree 4 mm Telescope	Bent suction	Antrum curette (round)
30-degree Wide-angle 4 mm telescope	Septum needle	Antrum curette (oblong)
70-degree Wide-angle 4 mm telescope	Freer elevator	Antrum curette (oval, size 1)
30-degree 2.7 mm Telescope	Antrum curette (forward cutting)	Antrum curette (oval, size 2)
	Antrum curette (backward cutting)	Antrum curette (oval, size 3)

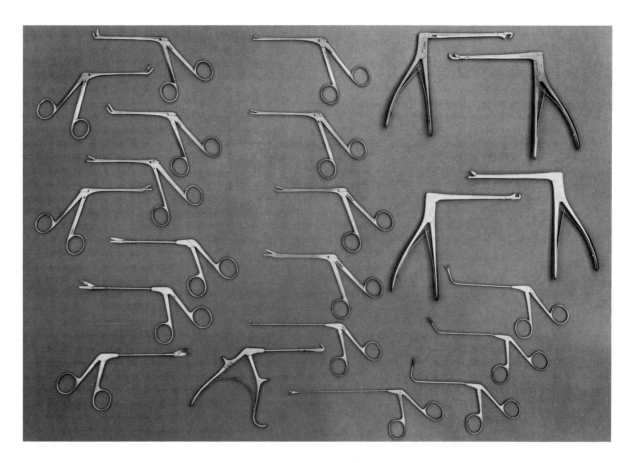

Figure 4.1E. Richard Wolf Medical Instruments endoscopic sinus surgery instruments.

90-degree Weil-Blakesley forceps (size 2)	Weil-Blakesley forceps (straight, size 1)	Sinus punch (retrograde, downward cutting)
Weil-Blakesley forceps (upturned, size 2)	Weil-Blakesley forceps (straight, size 2)	Sinus punch (60-degree upward cutting)
Weil-Blakesley forceps (upturned, size 3)	Takahashi forceps (size 2)	Sinus punch (straight cutting)
Weil-Blakesley forceps (straight, size 3)	Struychen nasal cutter	Sinus punch (90-degree upward cutting)
Weil-Blakesley forceps (straight, size 2)	Punch biopsy forceps (straight)	Double spoon forceps (70-degree angle, vertical cutting)
Turbinate scissors (straight)	Rice-Schaefer retrograde antrum punch	Double spoon forceps (70-degree angle, horizontal cutting)
Turbinate scissors (left)	Biopsy forceps	Double spoon forceps (100-degree angle, horizontal cutting)
Turbinate scissors (right)		

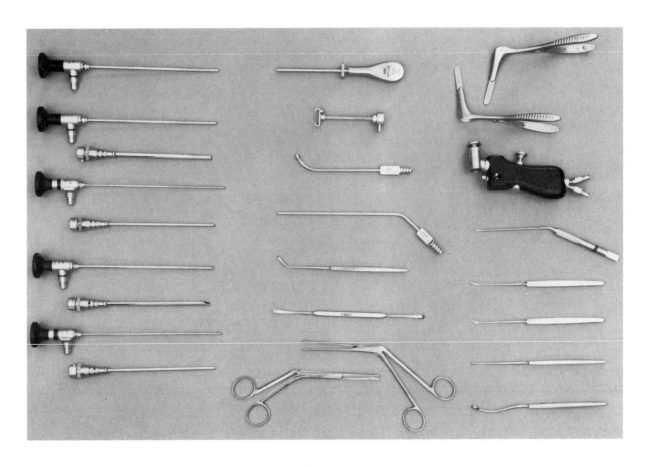

Figure 4.1F. Richard Wolf Medical Instruments (continued).

0-degree Wide-angle 4 mm telescope

25-degree Wide-angle 4 mm telescope

4 mm Suction-irrigation sheath (25 degree)

25-degree Wide-angle (Panoview plus) 4 mm telescope

4 mm Suction-irrigation sheath (25 degree)

70-degree Wide-angle 4 mm telescope

4 mm Suction-irrigation sheath (70 degree)

25-degree 2.7 mm Telescope

2.7 mm Suction-irrigation sheath (25 degree)

5 mm Trocar and cannula

Telescope bridge

4 mm Bent suction

4 mm Straight suction

Antrum curette (backward cutting)

Freer elevator

Packing forceps

Nasal scissors (straight)

Nasal speculum (right)

Nasal speculum (left)

Suction-irrigation handle

Bipolar nasal cautery

Sickle knife (blunt)

Sickle knife (pointed)

Antrum curette (round)

Antrum curette (oval, size 2)

Time should be allotted for adequate vasoconstriction and, if needed, anesthesia to permit maximal visualization of the nose when septal deflections compromise passage of a telescope. Cottonoids saturated with 4% lidocaine or cocaine may be placed at the site of obstruction to provide further anesthesia. The nose can then be examined, and one recommended routine is to initially advance the standard 30-degree or wide-angle 25- or 30-degree telescope along the floor of the nose. In this way, one can visualize the orifice of the nasolacrimal duct, inferolateral nasal wall, eustachian tube orifice and nasopharynx (Kennedy et al., 1985). The second passage of the endoscope is immediately inferior to the middle turbinate and provides viewing of the sphenoethmoid recess, middle meatus, and sphenoid ostium. Each of these sites may be variably difficult to examine because of the presence of polyps, degenerated mucous membrane, or pneumatization of the middle turbinate. The last passage of the telescope should be directed toward the frontal recess, thus crossing adjacent to the junction of the middle turbinate and the agger nasi cells.

Office Surgery

Such procedures as biopsy of the nose or sinuses, antral puncture, removal of several small or isolated large polyps, and control of epistaxis can be performed well in the office. All of these procedures require the cooperation of the patient and are enhanced by the skill of the physician in administering topical and infiltrative anesthesia. In the more extensive procedures, regional blocks, such as anesthetizing the sphenopalatine nerve, are particularly useful. In all procedures, the key to success is waiting 10 minutes or more after placement of the anesthetic agent to optimize its effect. The selection of further equipment to perform such procedures depends on the scope of the intended office surgery. As a minimum, we would recommend purchasing 45-degree Weil-Blakesley forceps, curved suction cannula, and if antral biopsies are to be performed, an antral trocar and forceps. Additional instruments, such as double spoon forceps, can be added to the office set as they are needed.

Antral Endoscopy

Endoscopic examination of the maxillary antrum is a simple procedure that can be performed well under local anesthesia and in an office setting. The antrostomy can be performed either at the canine fossa or beneath the inferior turbinate. However, we would recommend the former because visualization of the maxillary sinus is better and the procedure is simpler and well tolerated by the patient. When puncturing the canine fossa, anesthesia should first be topical (4% cocaine or lidocaine on a cotton pledget), followed by infiltration of the appropriate agent. A 5 mm trocar is introduced under sterile conditions through the anterior wall of the maxilla using a rotating action that takes advantage of the design of the trocar and minimizes thrusting the instrument through the sinus. After the trocar is within the sinus, the stylet is removed, and a 4 mm telescope is passed into the sheath of the trocar and the sinus is examined. Biopsies can be taken either by directing the trocar sheath under endoscopic control at the object of interest and then placing a forceps through the sheath or by using an optical forceps (telescope with attached forceps) passed through the sheath of the trocar. Whatever the method used, antral endoscopy is a valuable alternative to Caldwell-Luc or conventional antrostomies as a means to inspect the maxillary antrum and to biopsy suspicious lesions on radiographs.

EVALUATION OF THE SURGICAL PATIENT

The basic elements of the clinical evaluation of the patient with recurrent sinusitis or nasal polyps are the history, physical examination, and radiographs. A minimum of two of these elements must be abnormal before recommending surgical treatment.

History

The most important points of this part of the evaluation include previous pain or tenderness over the paranasal sinuses, mucopurulent rhinorrhea, and the response to prior medical management. Many patients associate any type of head pain with sinus disease. Patients with recurrent or chronic sinusitis (the difference between the two conditions is difficult to define) should be able to localize their pain or tenderness to the involved sinus. The sphenoid sinus is an exception to this statement in that pain may be referred to the vertex of the head. As sinus disease progresses, the pain may be no longer as well localized; for example, in advanced ethmoiditis, there may be retro-orbital pain. Mucopurulent rhinorrhea is another important physical finding because it is indicative of bacterial sinusitis, whereas clear nasal drainage suggests allergic disease (Figure 4.2).

The patient's response to previous medical management is very important because it provides a record of the adequacy of prior treatment and severity of the disease. Many patients believe that they have significant sinusitis when, in fact, they have received less than optimal therapy in the form of multiple courses of short-term (e.g., 5 days) antibiotics, often in inadequate doses. In our opinion, sinusitis refractory to medical management implies multiple episodes of bacterial sinusitis that either does not improve after 10 to 14 days of agents effective against the pneumococcus, *Haemophilus,* and staphylococci or repeated recurrence of disease shortly after completing a course of antibiotics. In the patient with polyps, the adequacy of prior immunotherapy must be evaluated before recommending surgery. Particularly in the younger patient, the physician should consider congenital disorders, such as cystic fibrosis or hypogammaglobulinemia, and look for concurrent lower respiratory tract disease as an indicator of broader illness. Finally, the past history of surgical procedures gives further insight into the severity and nature of the patient's problem.

The most common reason for patients to not improve significantly after multiple procedures is failure to exenterate the frontal recess and infundibular cells of the anterior ethmoid because of the difficulty in reaching this

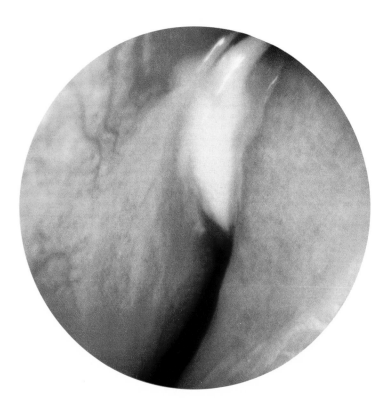

Figure 4.2. Mucopurulent drainage in middle meatus of left nose.

group of cells by more conventional procedures. Therefore, in recommending surgery, the history should both be consistent with sinusitis and demonstrate failure to improve after multiple trials of medical therapy.

Physical Examination

The physical examination should be directed toward confirming the history and looking for evidence of obstruction to the outflow of the sinuses into the nose. Such obstruction may include an isolated polyp in the middle meatus, a deviated septum compromising the ostiomeatal complex, or a concha bullosa pressing against the lateral wall of the nose (Figures 4.3, 4.4, 4.5, 5.12A). As disease progresses, the need for surgery becomes more apparent. For example, total obstruction of the nose by nasal polyps requires both medical and surgical treatment, with little hope for success using only one of these therapies.

To best prepare for surgical intervention, the physician needs to develop a routine for preoperatively visualizing the nose. Obviously, there should be as few surprises as possible in the operating room. The physician's routine should include viewing the ostiomeatal complex, the anterior wall of the sphenoid, the nasopharynx, and the frontal recess. The use of vasoconstrictive agents to optimize this examination is highly recommended. Following the physical examination, the physician should have a clearer understanding of the possible etiology of the patient's problem and the anatomy of that patient's nose.

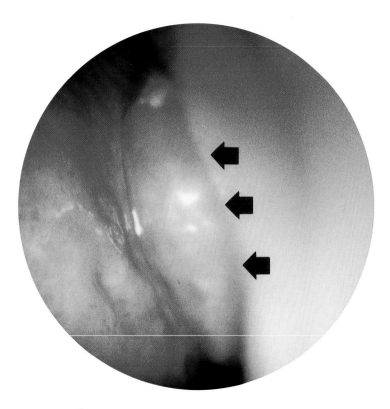

Figure 4.3. Polyp filling middle meatus of left nose (arrows).

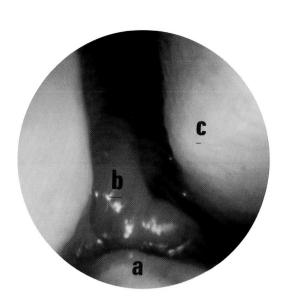

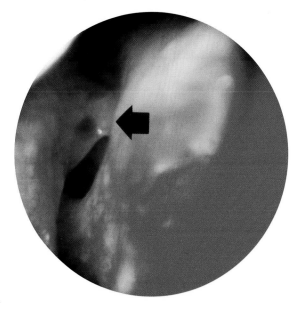

Figure 4.4. Inferior turbinate (a) is visualized with polyp superior (b) and middle turbinate lateral (c).

Figure 4.5. Spur (arrow) from left middle turbinate impinging on middle meatus, resulting in recurrent sinusitis.

Radiographs

Many physicians are rightfully concerned that advocates of endoscopic sinus surgery also have become proponents of CT scanning in a time of cost containment. In reality, a coronal CT scan of the paranasal sinuses may be far more cost-effective than repeated plain films and far more likely to aid in the treatment of that patient (Som et al., 1986 a, b). CT scanning shows precisely separate volumes of bone and soft tissue that may be the focus of infection, and such foci are frequently missed by plain film radiography. However, this does not mean that patients with one or two episodes of sinusitis require CT scanning. Once the focus or the extensiveness of disease has been delineated, the CT scan also serves as an important guide for the surgeon (Figure 4.6). Some of the important landmarks include (1) the proximity of the floor of the orbit to the potential location of the supra-inferior turbinate antrostomy, (2) the pneumatization of the ethmoid sinus, (3) the location of the natural ostium of the maxillary sinus, (4) the septation of the sphenoid sinus and the location of the internal carotid artery, and (5) the pneumatization and depth of the frontal sinus.

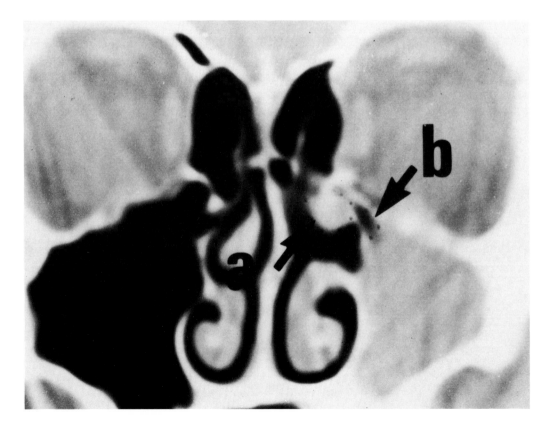

Figure 4.6. Coronal CT scan of 16-year-old female after extensive antibiotic therapy for orbital cellulitis secondary to sinusitis. Scan shows paradoxical middle turbinate (a) obstructing outflow of maxillary infundibulum (b).

OPERATIVE EQUIPMENT SELECTION

The novice endoscopic surgeon is fortunate today to be able to choose among several excellent instrument manufacturers. The principal differences in the major optical companies reflect the philosophies of the surgeons who worked with these companies to develop equipment to best perform their particular surgical procedures. Many of these differences are more perceived than real. Those that are real concern the choice of telescopes and the use of suction irrigation, with the rest of the hardware being very similar.

Optical Telescopes

In selecting a sinus endoscope, one must consider the optical axis, degrees of vision, and resolution at the visual periphery of the telescope. The optical axis refers to the center of vision, and telescopes are designated by this axis. The degrees of vision is a measure of the actual size of the visual field of the instrument. For example, one endoscope may be a wide-angle 30-degree telescope and the other a standard 45-degree telescope, but the former instrument's field of vision eclipses the field of the latter. However, the former telescope is only as useful as the skill of the optical manufacture in minimizing distortion at the visual periphery. To assist the reader in evaluating these different types of optical telescopes, we constructed a 4-inch-diameter sphere as a bench test. Each telescope was placed in the center of the sphere, and a photograph was taken through the endoscope (Figure 4.7). This helps illustrate that there are two basic choices that can be made; either use two wide-angle telescopes (25-degree or 30-degree and 70-degree) or four standard telescopes (0-degree, 30-degree, 70-degree, and 90-degree or 120-degree). The physician should evaluate these systems and decide which he or she prefers.

Figure 4.7. Bench test of endoscopes. 0° indicates portion of sphere 2 inches directly in front of telescope, 90° is in reference to 0° and 2 inches above the tip of the telescope, and arrow points toward 0°. An artifact from the testing procedure, not the telescopes, appears in some figures to the right of the 0° marker.

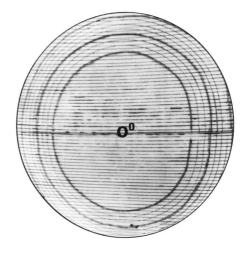

Figure 4.7A. Richards 0-degree wide-angle 4 mm telescope.

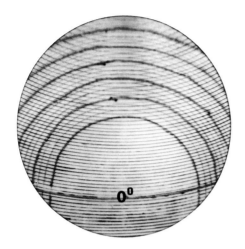

Figure 4.7B. Richards 25-degree wide-angle 4 mm telescope.

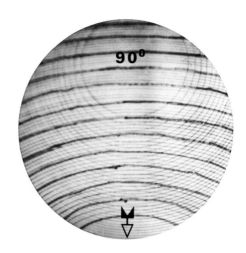

Figure 4.7C. Richards 70-degree wide-angle 4 mm telescope.

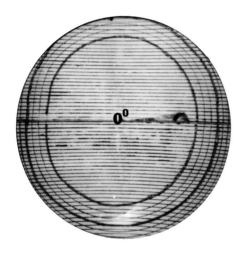

Figure 4.7D. Storz 0-degree 4 mm telescope.

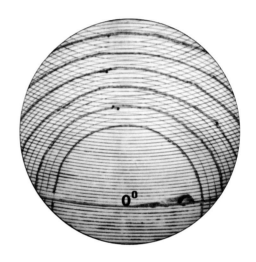

Figure 4.7E. Storz 30-degree 4 mm telescope.

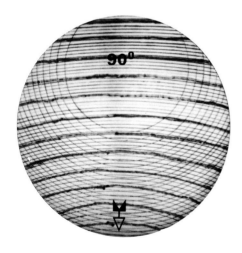

Figure 4.7F. Storz 70-degree 4 mm telescope.

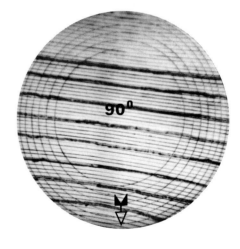

Figure 4.7G. Storz 90-degree 4 mm telescope.

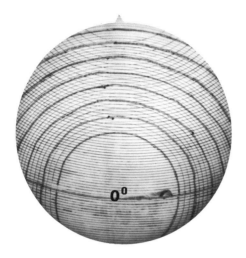

Figure 4.7H. Storz 30-degree wide-angle 4 mm telescope.

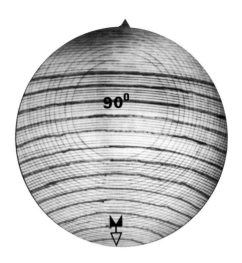

Figure 4.7I. Storz 70-degree wide-angle 4 mm telescope.

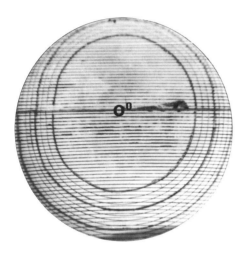

Figure 4.7J. Wolf 0-degree wide-angle 4 mm telescope.

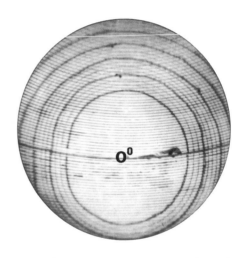

Figure 4.7K. Wolf 25-degree wide-angle 4 mm telescope.

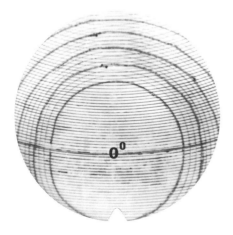

Figure 4.7L. Wolf 25-degree wide-angle (Panoview plus) 4 mm telescope.

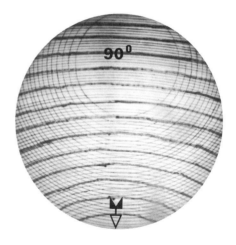

Figure 4.7M. Wolf 70-degree wide-angle 4 mm telescope.

Suction Irrigation

This device consists of a telescope sheath coupled to a handle. The purpose of suction irrigation is to prevent fogging of the endoscope by continuously drawing air past the telescope and to remove blood on the lens via irrigation. If the suction irrigator does not do both of these tasks well, it is not worth purchasing. This instrument is not a prerequisite to performing endoscopic sinus surgery, and the sheath does slightly limit access to the operative field in the narrow nose. Fogging can be minimized by periodic warming of the telescope in hot water or by placing this instrument against the buccal mucous membrane. However, the more extensive the surgical procedure, the more useful is suction irrigation, particularly in avoiding the need to clean the lens of the telescope frequently.

Hardware

Of the various forceps manufactured, the 45-degree or upturned and 90-degree Weil-Blakesley (or Blakesley-Wilde) are the most useful. A retrograde antrum punch (sideward and backward cutting) forceps is helpful in enlarging the natural ostium of the maxillary sinus, and the double spoon forceps are invaluable in removing tissue from the frontal and maxillary sinuses. A bent suction provides a means of aspirating blood and secretions from the ethmoid, frontal, and maxillary sinuses. Finally, the coupling of suction to the Blakesley forceps is particularly useful. The rest of the sinus equipment armamentarium depends on both the practice and the budget of the surgeon. In a teaching hospital, an endoscopic camera is practically a necessity and can be likened to a sidearm on the operating microscope.

LITERATURE CITED

Kennedy, D. W., Zinreich, J., Rosenbaum, A. E., and Johns, M. E.
1985 Functional endoscopic sinus surgery. *Arch. Otolaryngol.,* 111:576–582.
Som, P. M., Lawson, W., Biller, H. F., and Lanzieri, C. F.
1986a Ethmoid sinus disease: CT evaluation in 400 cases. Part I. Nonsurgical patients. *Radiology,* 159:591–597.
Som, P. M., Lawson, W., Biller, H. F., Lanzieri, C. F., Sachdev, V. P., and Rigamonti, D.
1986b Ethmoid sinus disease: CT evaluation in 400 cases. Part III. Craniofacial resection. *Radiology,* 159:605–612.

5

Functional Endoscopic
Paranasal Sinus Surgery

The Technique of Messerklinger

INDICATIONS

Functional endoscopic sinus surgery is based on two principles. First, obstruction in the anterior ethmoid may block the maxillary, frontal, and posterior ethmoid sinuses and, on occasion, the sphenoid sinus and eustachian tube. Stated another way, persistent disease in one of these sinuses is most likely due to undiagnosed, untreated anterior ethmoid disease (Messerklinger, 1985). Second, relief of obstruction in the anterior ethmoids may allow the other sinuses to drain and return to normal. The maxillary sinus ostium, in particular, lies in a gutter where the purulent drainage from the ethmoids will pour across it. It is implied in this concept that the mucosal disease is reversible with adequate drainage (Stammberger, 1985).

This technique is indicated whenever adequate medical management has failed in bacterial sinusitis. It is the first intervention of choice, and the technique often gives good results with minimum morbidity and rapid recovery.

CONTRAINDICATIONS

There are probably no absolute contraindications to this technique other than complicated frontal sinusitis, when more traditional techniques should be used. Certainly, this approach would be inadequate for frontal sinusitis with an epidural or subdural abscess. A relative contraindication, particularly in inexperienced hands, would be ethmoiditis with an orbital complication. Extensive recurrent or chronic disease is probably better managed by a total sphenoethmoidectomy.

CASE HISTORY

A 42-year-old woman had a 5-year history of recurrent right maxillary sinusitis. She had undergone numerous courses of antibiotics. With each course, the facial pain and mucopurulent rhinorrhea would eventually stop, only to recur within a few weeks. Two separate antral windows with irrigations failed.

Rhinoscopy revealed mucopurulent rhinorrhea coming from the middle meatus. The remainder of the physical examination was normal. CT scan (Figure 5.1A) revealed a completely opacified right maxillary sinus with obvious obstruction at the ostiomeatal unit.

The patient underwent right endoscopic sinus surgery with removal of the uncinate process and bulla ethmoidalis. On completion of this, the opening to the maxillary sinus could be seen easily and was of adequate size not needing to be enlarged. The patient did well postoperatively, and a CT scan (Figure 5.1B) showed complete clearing of the right maxillary sinus and an open ostiomeatal unit.

INSTRUMENTATION

Richards, Karl Storz, and Richard Wolf make instruments that serve admirably for this operative technique (*see* Figure 4.1). The telescopes come in different diameters and different optical axes. Most of the work in this technique can be performed with the 0-degree, 30-degree, and 70-degree or wide-angle 25-degree or 30-degree and 70-degree telescopes in 4 mm diameter. Much of the dissection can be performed with the 45-degree Weil-Blakesley forcep. The straight biting, 90-degree, and reverse biting forceps are frequently useful.

ANESTHESIA

Functional sinus surgery can be performed under local or general anesthesia, depending on the preference of the surgeon and the patient. In either case, thorough vasoconstriction is imperative. This may be started in the preanesthetic holding area with Afrin or some other vasoconstrictive spray. In the operating room, the nasal cavity should be packed with cottonoids, soaked (but wrung out) in 1% lidocaine with 1:100,000 epinephrine. After 5 minutes, the cottonoid pledgets should be removed, and the middle turbinate and middle meatus should be injected with 1% lidocaine with 1:100,000 epinephrine. For this technique, no more than 3 ml to 5 ml are needed per side. If there are significant polyps, they may be removed at this time in the traditional fashion with a headlight.

Figure 5.1A. Preoperative CT scan showing chronic maxillary sinusitis with complete obstruction of the ostiomeatal unit.

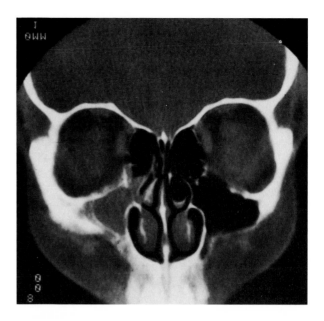

Figure 5.1B. Postoperative CT scan of same patient in Figure 5.1A. Note resolution of the maxillary sinus disease and the open ostiomeatal unit.

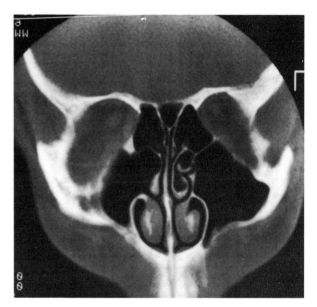

If a septoplasty is needed to gain access with the instruments, it should be performed first. Theoretically, elective septoplasty should be postponed to avoid exposing the septal cartilage to infection. In practice, however, this does not seem to be a problem. After the injection, the nasal cavity should be repacked with soaked cottonoids, with care being taken to place one cottonoid into the middle meatus. Another 5 minutes should be allowed to elapse, during which prepping and draping can be done. However, the entire operation is performed on infected tissue in a grossly contaminated intranasal field. It seems analogous to prepping and draping to drain a neck abscess.

OPERATIVE TECHNIQUE

Step 1   (Illustrated on pages 80–81)

Once the nasal mucosa is thoroughly vasoconstricted, a complete examination should be performed. This is best done with the 0-degree or wide-angle 25-degree or 30-degree telescope and should be performed gently to avoid tearing the mucosa and causing annoying bleeding. The nasal cavity should be examined systematically, with particular attention being paid to the middle meatus (Figures 5.2 A,B, 6.2C), and any other area of abnormality on the CT scan.

Step 2   (Illustrated on pages 82–83)

The initial maneuver is to open the anterior ethmoid air cells within the uncinate process, which is generally immediately lateral to the anterior middle turbinate. This can be performed most elegantly by making an incision with the sickle knife or Cottle elevator (Figure 5.3C) and spreading the mucosa medially. Blakesley or Takahashi forceps can then be inserted so that one jaw is in the incision and one jaw is in the middle meatus (Figure 5.3A). The tissue between the jaws (the uncinate process) is grasped and removed. This should establish the initial correct plane of dissection. Bear in mind that the ethmoids are approximately 0.5 cm wide in this region.

Step 3   (Illustrated on pages 84–87)

Next the forceps should be used to remove the remainder of the area from the fovea superiorly to the insertion of the inferior turbinate inferiorly. The dissection then proceeds posteriorly across the hiatus semilunaris into the bulla ethmoidalis (Figures 5.4A, B, C). The bulla is treated similarly to the uncinate (Figures 5.5A, B, C, 5.6A, B, C).

Step 4   (Illustrated on pages 88–91)

At this point, the operation would be completed if there were no sinus disease other than the anterior ethmoids (Figure 5.6C). Usually, however, this is not the case. Most commonly, there is also maxillary sinus disease, and in that situation, the next step is to identify the natural ostium. Usually, this cannot be identified earlier in the procedure but often becomes visible as the inferior aspect of the uncinate and bulla are widely opened. If the natural ostium seems patent at this point, nothing further need be done. If it is not or if it is in question, it should be enlarged anteriorly using the reverse biting forceps or posteriorly with the straight forceps until it is 1.5 cm to 2.0 cm in diameter (Figures 5.7A, B, C).

Occasionally, even after seeming completion of the anterior ethmoid dissection, the natural ostium will not be visible because of mucosal hypertrophy. It can be found by palpating just above the inferior turbinate approximately halfway between its anterior and posterior ends in the membranous meatus. Care should be taken to avoid angling superiorly to avoid injury to the orbit. Gentle removal of mucosa with the 90-degree Weil-Blakesley forceps in this location will usually uncover the natural ostium, which should then be enlarged (Figure 5.7D). If the patient's problem is ostiomeatal complex disease alone, nothing further need be done.

ADDITIONAL MANEUVERS

Step 5: Posterior Ethmoid Disease   (Illustrated on pages 92–93)

If the patient also has posterior ethmoid disease, further dissection is indicated. At the completion of the preceding steps, the posterior limit of the operative field should be the basal (ground) lamella (Figure 5.6A). This bony partition extends from the middle turbinate to the lamina papyracea and separates the anterior from the posterior ethmoid air cells. This partition should be penetrated and the posterior cells entered. From this approach, a complete ethmoidectomy can be performed, stopping at the anterior wall of the sphenoid (Figures 5.8A, B, C). Care should be taken laterally and superiorly because of the changing relationships to the orbit and to the anterior cranial fossa.

Step 6: Sphenoid Disease   (Illustrated on pages 94–95)

Should there also be sphenoid disease, the sphenoid can be entered after completion of the posterior ethmoidectomy (Figures 5.9A, B). The natural ostium usually can be identified and then enlarged in an inferior and medial direction. It is probably not wise to enlarge the ostium superiorly or laterally. If the natural ostium cannot be identified, the anterior wall of the sinus may be entered and the opening enlarged (Figure 5.9C).

Step 7: Frontal Sinus Disease   (Illustrated on pages 96–99)

In patients with frontal sinus disease, an additional step is required. The superior-anterior ethmoid air cells in the frontal recess area must be opened, and the nasofrontal duct or ostium must be cleared of obstruction (Figures 5.10A, B, C). This must be performed with an angled telescope to adequately visualize the area to ensure complete clearing of the duct. Thorough removal of these air cells is essential to ensure continued adequate drainage.

On occasion, it may be necessary to enter the frontal sinus. Specially curved forceps are available for this purpose. If need be, the duct can be enlarged all the way into the sinus, this step is rarely necessary (Figures 5.11A, B, C).

Figure 5.2. Step 1.

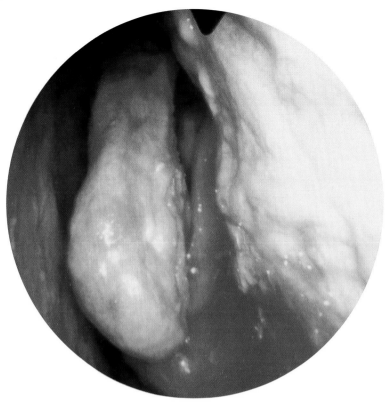

Figure 5.2A. Endoscopic view of middle meatus on left showing the middle turbinate medially, the bulge of the uncinate anteriorly, and the bulla ethmoidalis behind.

Step 8: Concha Bullosa   (Illustrated on page 100)

An air cell within the middle turbinate will need to be opened if (1) it is diseased or (2) it has expanded the turbinate so that the lateral aspect encroaches on the middle meatus. This is best managed by entering the air cell at the anterior end of the middle turbinate with a sickle knife or the biting forceps (Figure 5.12A). After this, the lateral wall is removed sufficiently to establish adequate drainage and adequately enlarge the middle meatus (Figure 5.12B). When this is necessary, great care must be taken postoperatively to prevent adhesions between the middle turbinate and the lateral nasal wall.

Step 9: Maxillary Sinus Pathology

If the disease in the maxillary sinus consists of edematous mucosa, polyps, and retention cysts, establishing adequate drainage through the natural os-

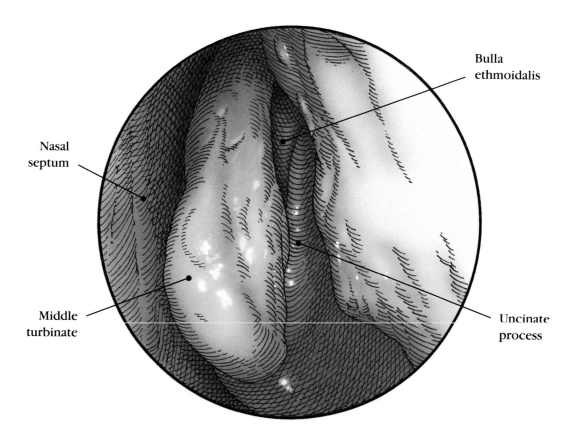

Figure 5.2B. Artist's illustration of Figure 5.2A.

tium generally will allow the mucosa to return to normal over time. Occasionally, there will be disease that requires direct manipulation (e.g., pyocele, lesion that needs to be biopsied). Depending on location, this can be done in one of two ways. If routine endoscopic sinus surgery also has been required, the goal probably can be accomplished transnasally. Once the natural ostium has been enlarged, a nasoantral window can be created through the inferior meatus. The maxillary sinus can be observed with the telescope through one opening while the forceps or curette is inserted through the other.

If only the maxillary sinus is the problem, a canine fossa puncture can be performed with the trocar. The lesion can be identified by inserting the telescope through the trocar sheath. The sheath is then pointed directly at the lesion, the telescope is removed, the forceps are inserted, and the tissue removed. If necessary, the optical forceps can be used through the sheath.

Figure 5.3. Step 2.
5.3A

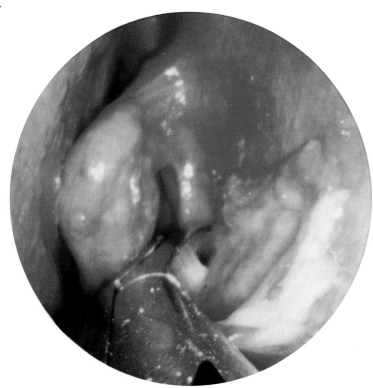

Figure 5.3A. Endoscopic view of Weil-Blakesley 45-degree forceps resecting uncinate process.

Figure 5.3B. Artist's illustration of Figure 5.3A.

Figure 5.3C. Sagittal photograph with Cottle elevator incising anterior aspect of uncinate process. This also can be done with the sickle knife. Opening the uncinate is the initial step in beginning its resection.

5.3B

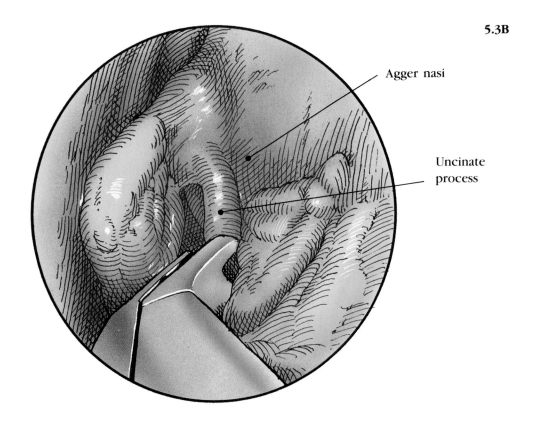

Agger nasi

Uncinate process

5.3C

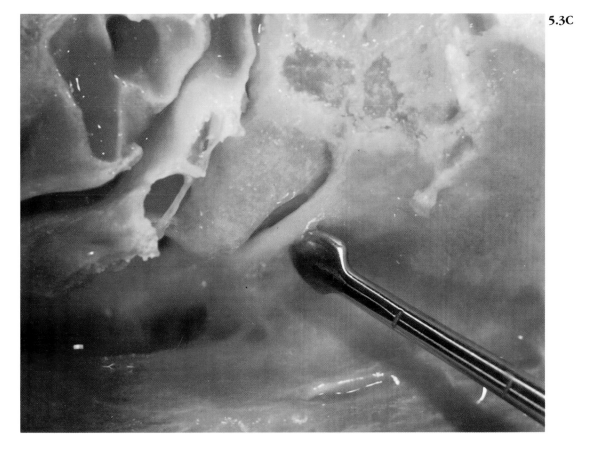

Figure 5.4. Step 3.
5.4A

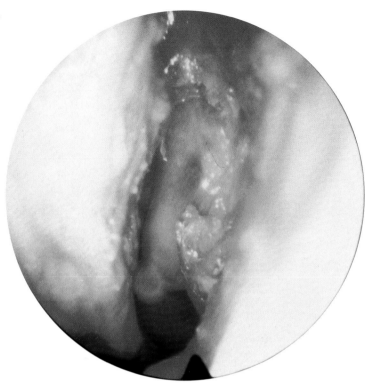

Figure 5.4A. Endoscopic view with uncinate process removed and bulla ethmoidalis ahead. The bulla is the next structure removed.

Figure 5.4B. Illustration shows bulla ethmoidalis with the resected uncinate process anterior and to the patient's left of the bulla.

Figure 5.4C. Sagittal view with 45-degree Weil-Blakesley forceps entering bulla ethmoidalis after uncinate process has been removed.

5.4B

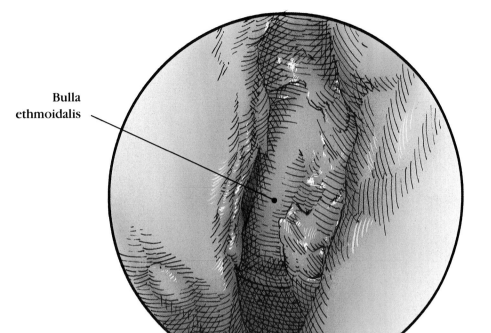

Bulla
ethmoidalis

5.4C

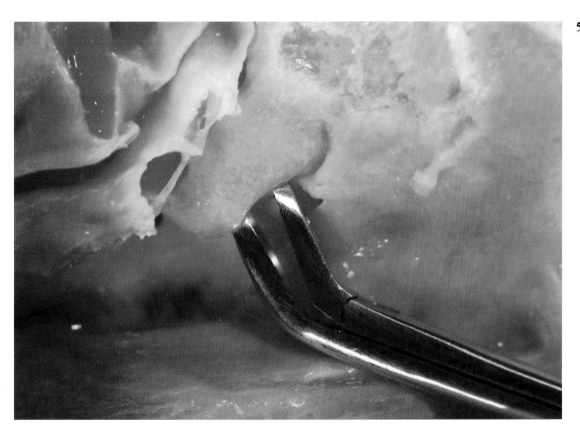

Figure 5.5. Step 3.

5.5A

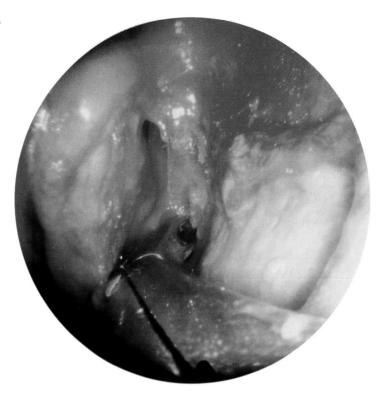

Figure 5.5A. Endoscopic view of 45-degree Weil-Blakesley forceps within bulla ethmoidalis.

Figure 5.5B. Artist's illustration of Figure 5.5A.

Figure 5.5C. Sagittal view showing Weil-Blakesley forceps having removed bulla ethmoidalis.

5.5B

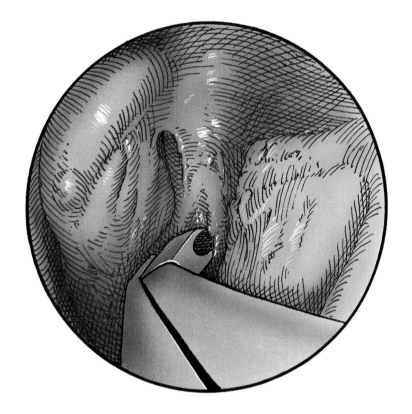

5.5C

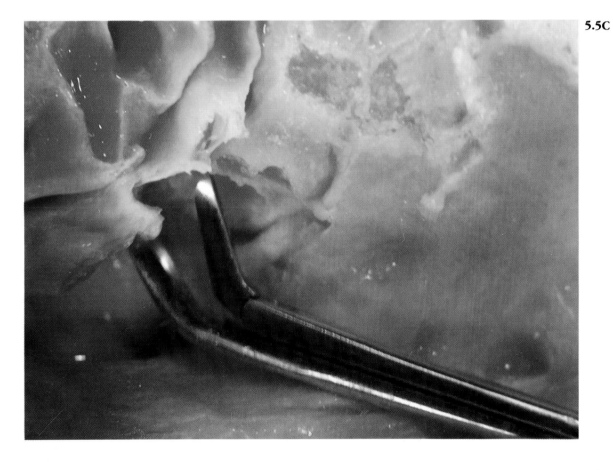

Figure 5.6. Step 4.

5.6A

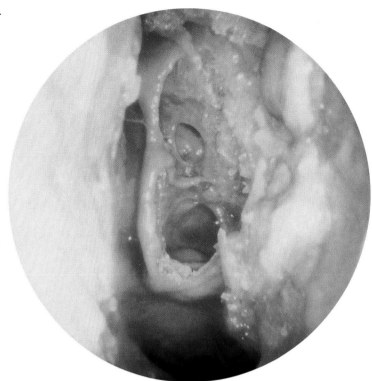

Figure 5.6A. Endoscopic view with uncinate process and bulla ethmoidalis removed and basal (ground) lamella in clear view.

Figure 5.6B. Artist's illustration of Figure 5.6A.

Figure 5.6C. Sagittal view showing 45-degree Weil-Blakesley forceps in posterior ethmoid cells after perforating the basal lamella.

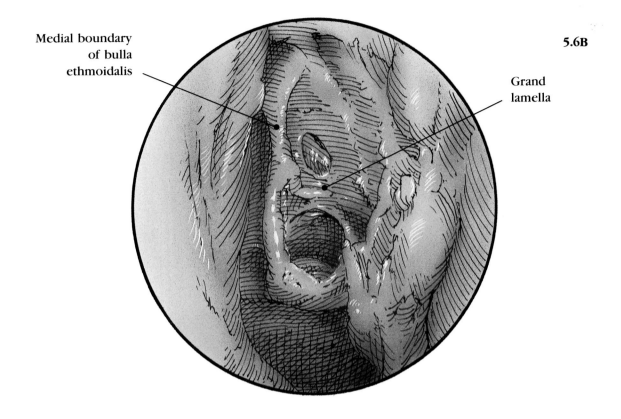

Medial boundary
of bulla
ethmoidalis

5.6B

Grand
lamella

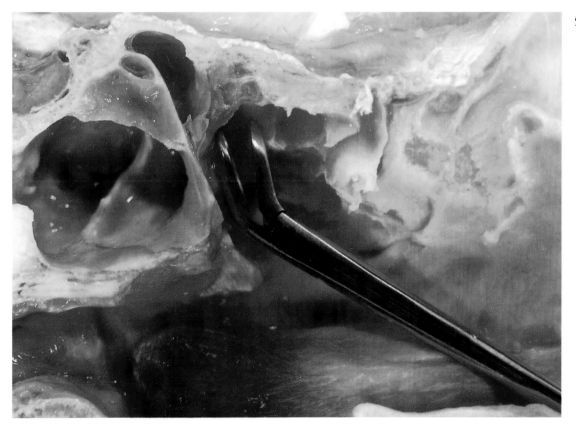

5.6C

Figure 5.7. Step 4.

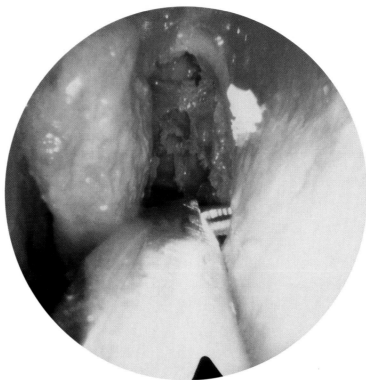

Figure 5.7A. Endoscopic view showing retrograde forceps in natural ostium of maxillary sinus. Posterior to the forceps are the posterior ethmoid cells. Medial to the forceps is the middle turbinate.

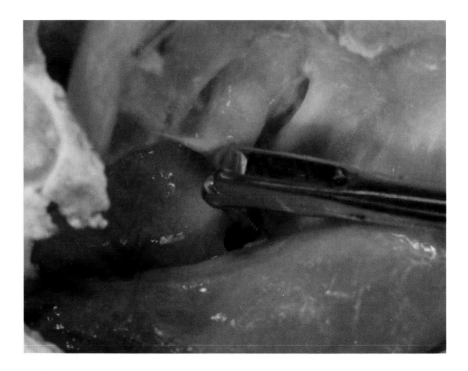

Figure 5.7B. Sagittal view showing retrograde forceps opening the natural ostium of the maxillary sinus.

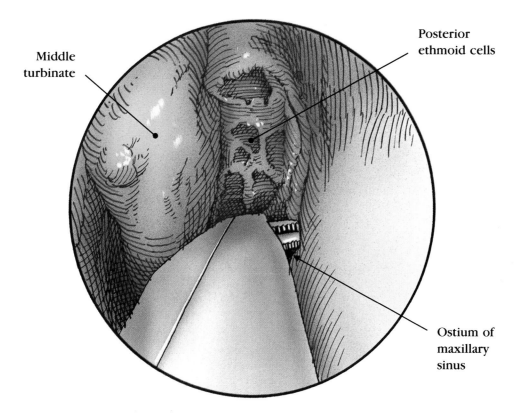

Middle turbinate

Posterior ethmoid cells

Ostium of maxillary sinus

Figure 5.7C. Artist's illustration of Figure 5.7A.

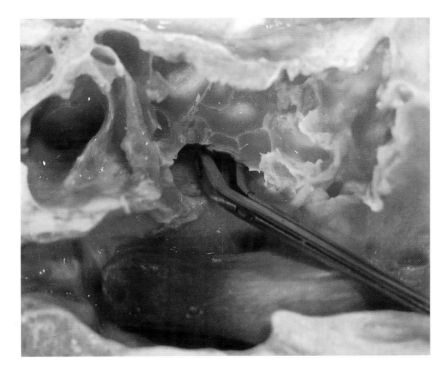

Figure 5.7D. Weil-Blakesley forceps enlarging maxillary sinus ostium.

Figure 5.8. Step 5.

5.8A

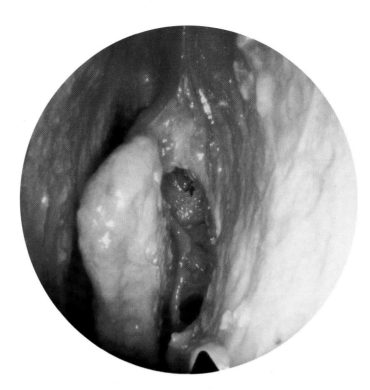

Figure 5.8A. Endoscopic view showing posterior ethmoid cells removed. Sphenoid sinus ostia is visible in lower part of photograph.

Figure 5.8B. Artist's illustration of Figure 5.8A.

Figure 5.8C. Sagittal view showing 45-degree Weil-Blakesley forceps in anterior aspect of ethmoid sinus after all cells of this sinus have been removed.

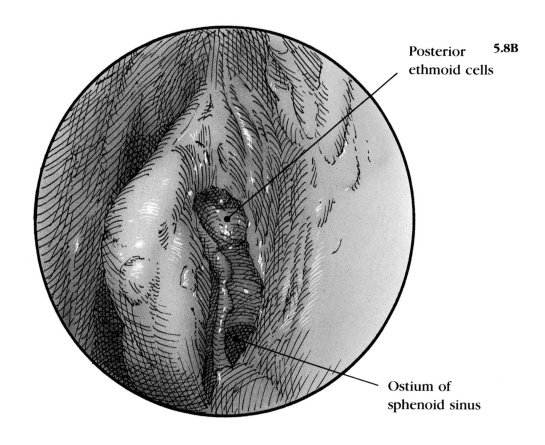

Posterior
ethmoid cells

5.8B

Ostium of
sphenoid sinus

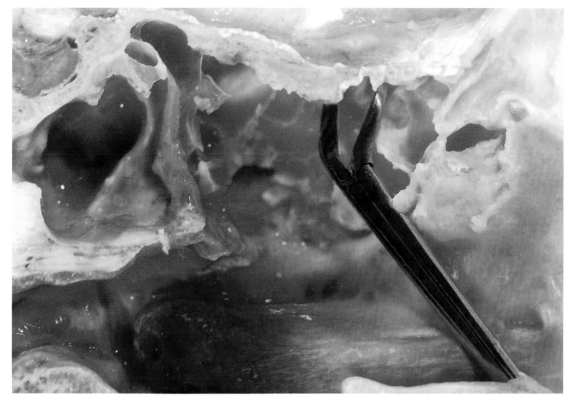

5.8C

Figure 5.9. Step 6.
5.9A

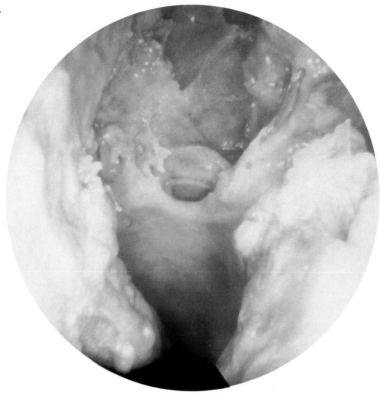

Figure 5.9A. Endoscopic view with posterior ethmoids removed and ostium of sphenoid sinus in middle of photograph.

Figure 5.9B. Artist's illustration of Figure 5.9A.

Figure 5.9C. Sagittal view of 45-degree Weil-Blakesley forceps within sphenoid sinus after complete ethmoidectomy.

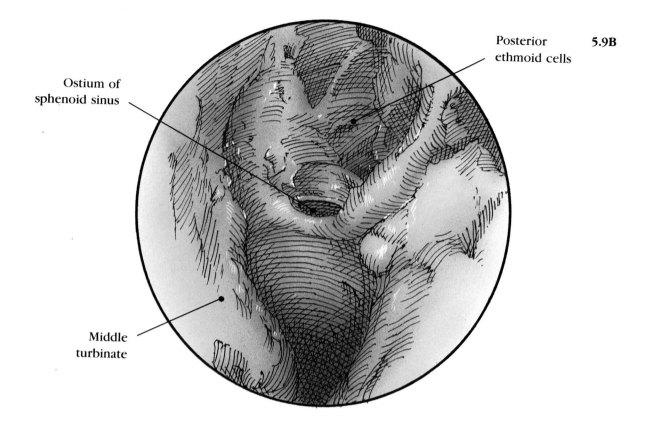

Ostium of
sphenoid sinus

Posterior
ethmoid cells

5.9B

Middle
turbinate

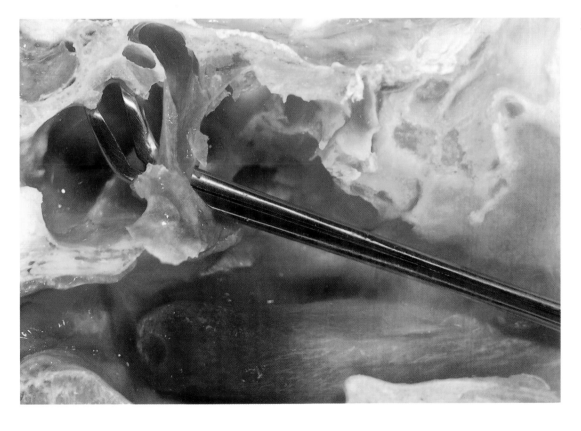

5.9C

Figure 5.10. Step 7.

5.10A

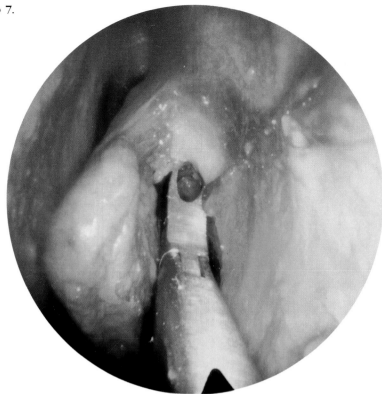

Figure 5.10A. Endoscopic view showing 45-degree Weil-Blakesley forceps resecting frontal recess cells to clear nasofrontal duct.

Figure 5.10B. Agger nasi cells have been partially removed to facilitate visualization of the frontal recess.

Figure 5.10C. Sagittal view with 45-degree forceps resecting frontal recess cells after completion of ethmoidectomy.

5.10B

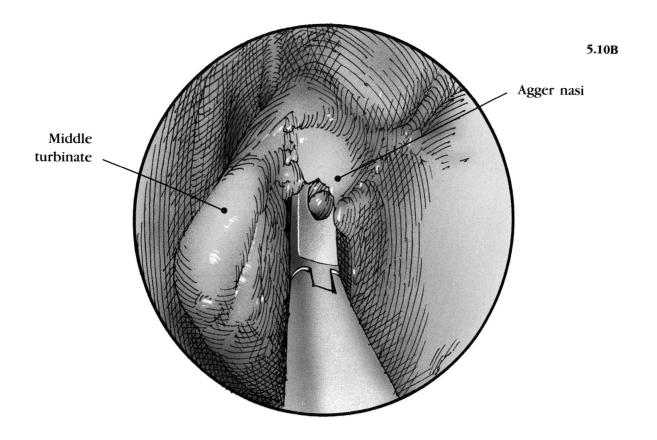

Middle turbinate

Agger nasi

5.10C

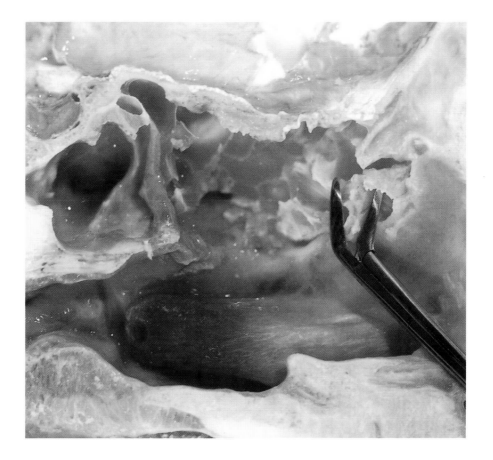

Figure 5.11. Step 7.
5.11A

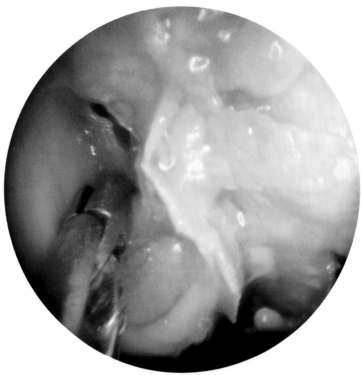

Figure 5.11A. Endoscopic view showing double spoon forceps in frontal recess with natural ostium of frontal sinus immediately superior to forceps.

Figure 5.11B. Artist's illustration of Figure 5.11A.

Figure 5.11C. Sagittal view showing double spoon forceps in frontal recess area after removal of agger nasi and frontal recess cells.

Frontal recess

Ostium of
frontal sinus

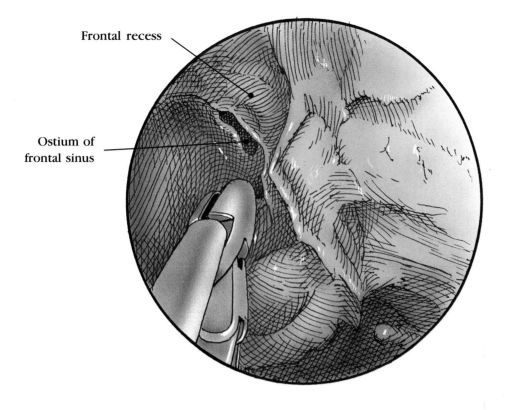

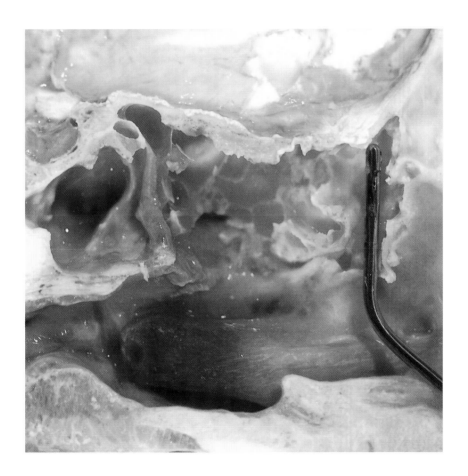

Figure 5.12. Step 8.

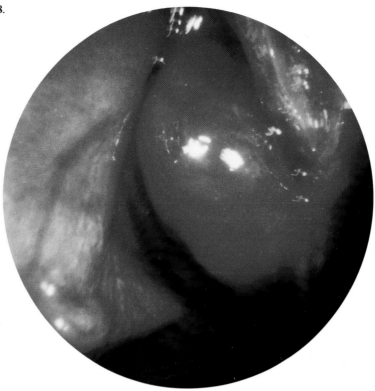

Figure 5.12A. Endoscopic view of concha bullosa of right nasal cavity.

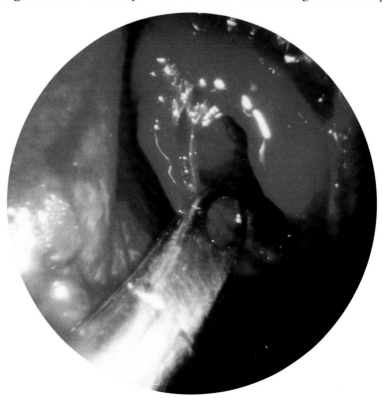

Figure 5.12B. Endoscopic view showing concha bullosa transected in the sagittal plane. Forceps are positioned to remove the lateral portion of the turbinate.

HIGHLIGHTS

1. This procedure is most useful in the patient with chronic recurrent or refractory sinusitis when the anterior ethmoids are involved.

2. For most patients, it is probably the logical first invasive procedure.

3. This technique does not alter the nasal response to allergies in those patients who have them.

4. Care should be taken to avoid denuding the middle turbinate.

5. Opening agger nasi cells aids in postoperative cleansing and evaluation.

6. In patients with a narrow middle meatus but no concha bullosa, it may be advisable to resect part of the anterior, hanging end of the middle turbinate.

POSTOPERATIVE CARE

Success in endoscopic sinus surgery requires more than performing the procedure correctly. Proper postoperative care is essential, and inadequate attention to detail can lead to failure. The objective is to keep the sinuses open and draining and to prevent scarring, which might subsequently occlude the ostia.

At the conclusion of the procedure, something should be done to minimize bleeding and crusting. Traditional gauze packing or Telfa gauze coated with an antibiotic ointment can be used. A third choice is to fill the operative site with an antibiotic ointment.

In the early postoperative period, the cavity should be inspected, and any clots or crusts should be removed. The patient should then begin nasal irrigations to keep the operative site clear. Considerable drainage should be expected and may continue several weeks. Irrigations should be performed as often as necessary to keep the site free of clots and crusts. This may be done effectively with a Grossan nasal irrigator attached to a Water Pik or a rubber bulb syringe and continued until healing is complete. Postirrigation application of a steroid nasal spray appears to aid healing, as does a 5- to 7-day course of antibiotics. Despite all this, excessive scarring may occur.

Complications

In the standard, unmodified Messerklinger technique, complications should be few and usually minor. Dissection too superiorly can lead to a cerebrospinal fluid leak. If this is recognized intraoperatively, it should be repaired endoscopically with fascia and tissue glue, with a mucosal flap if possible. If it is recognized postoperatively, conservative treatment should be instituted unless it is clearly too large to seal. If closure does not occur within 4 to 6 weeks, operative closure should be performed. Depending on the location and size, this may be done endoscopically or externally.

Dissection too laterally may lead to a breech of the lamina papyracea. The CT scan should be studied carefully preoperatively. Approximately 10% of people have an incomplete lamina papyracea. In addition, if previous ethmoid procedures have been performed, the lamina may have suffered an asymptomatic injury. If orbital fat is encountered, dissection should stop immediately in that area. Packing should not be used. If the injury is minimal, the patient can be expected to have some ecchymosis of the medial canthal area and lower eyelid, which will resolve in several days. Anything further demands an immediate ophthalmologic evaluation.

Dissection in the posterior ethmoids and sphenoid is more dangerous and is discussed in Chapter 6.

Dissection too anteriorly can lead to damage to the nasolacrimal apparatus. The bone around the lacrimal sac and the nasolacrimal duct is usually more dense, and this serves as a warning. However, even if either structure were injured, it would probably heal spontaneously. If epiphora persists, an intranasal endoscopic dacryocystorhinostomy can be performed (Rice, 1987).

It is possible also to damage the medial wall or floor of the orbit when exploring or enlarging the natural ostium of the maxillary sinus. Careful study of the preoperative CT scan will show the proximity of the orbit to the area of the natural ostium. In general, the orbit is closer anteriorly than posteriorly, and the search for the ostium should begin more posteriorly when it cannot be seen readily. In this situation, careful palpation usually will identify the ostium. Regardless, the instrument should always be advanced in an inferolateral direction and never superiorly.

LITERATURE CITED

Messerklinger W.
    1985 Endoskopische diagnose und chirurgie der rezidivierenden sinusitis. In: *Advances in Nose and Sinus Surgery,* edited by Z. Krajina, Zagreb University, Zagreb, Yugoslavia.
Rice, D. H.
    1987 Endoscopic intranasal dacryocysto-rhinostomy. Presented at the American Academy of Otolaryngology–Head and Neck Surgery Annual Meeting.
Stammberger H.
    1985 Endoscopic surgery for mycotic and chronic recurring sinusitis. *Ann. Otol. Rhinol. Laryngol.* (Suppl) 119:1–11.
Stammberger H.
    1986 Endoscopic endonasal surgery—concepts in treatment of recurring rhinosinusitis. Part II. Surgical technique. *Otolaryngol. Head Neck Surg.* 94:147–156.

6

Total Endoscopic Sphenoethmoidectomy
The Technique of Wigand

INDICATIONS

Total sphenoethmoidectomy is reserved for the patient with sinusitis or polyps extensively involving (i.e., a minimum of the ethmoid, sphenoid and maxillary sinuses) the ipsilateral or bilateral paranasal sinuses. This is a particularly safe procedure in the patient with significant disease who no longer has conventional landmarks (i.e., middle turbinate) as a result of previous surgery. The technique is specifically intended to permit the surgeon to progress from the sphenoid sinus anteriorly to exenterate the ethmoid sinus, using the fovea ethmoidalis as the superior boundary of the dissection (Wigand, 1981; Wigand et al., 1978).

CONTRAINDICATIONS

There are no contraindications in the otherwise healthy patient, as long as the disease process is confined to the paranasal sinuses.

CASE HISTORY

A 32-year-old female was referred with a 10-year history of repeated episodes of facial pain, mucopurulent rhinorrhea, nasal airway obstruction, and polyps. Previous medical management included immunotherapy, nasal steroids, and numerous courses of antibiotics during episodes of acute sinusitis. Previous surgical management included bilateral Caldwell-Luc procedures and intranasal ethmoidectomies 4 years previously. Physical examination revealed total obstruction of both nasal cavities with polyps, which precluded endoscopic visualization of the lateral nasal wall. CT scanning showed extensive disease of the paranasal sinuses (Figures 6.1A, B).

Operative management consisted of bilateral intranasal endoscopic sphenoethmoidectomies, frontal sinusotomies, and supra-inferior turbinate antrostomies. At surgery, the sinuses were filled with both polyps and dense, inspissated secretions. The postoperative course was unremarkable, and the patient returned to work within a week of surgery. Follow-up care has included nasal steroids and frequent endoscopic examination of the sinuses to observe for regrowth of polyps.

INSTRUMENTATION

A variety of endoscopes are available that may be used to perform the Wigand total sphenoethmoidectomy. Figure 4.1 shows equipment manufactured by three companies. Several instruments are particularly useful for this technique. First, a suction irrigation system is beneficial in dealing with increased bleeding that can occur in this more extensive surgical approach.

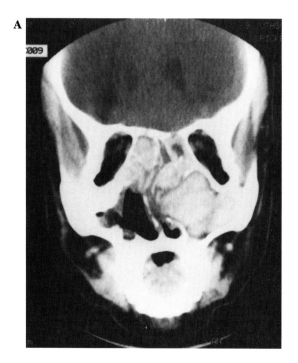
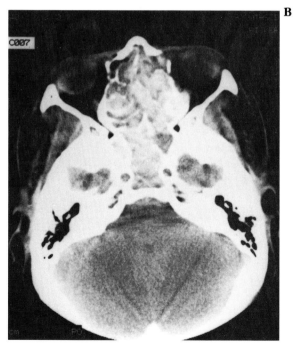

Figure 6.1A,B. Coronal **(A)** and axial **(B)** CT scans of a 32-year-old female with extensive nasal polyps. Note that the polyps were both of long duration and sufficient size to displace the nasal septum and show areas of neocalcification.

The effectiveness of this device is enhanced by placing the irrigation fluid under pressure by using a blood pressure pump. Second, forceps (known as double spoon forceps manufactured at various angles) have been developed specifically to permit the removal of tissue within the recesses of both the maxillary and frontal sinuses. Finally, sinus punch forceps are useful for both sphenoidotomy and frontal sinusotomy. In some cases, similar instruments can be found that will serve the same function, such as the use of the universal handle and its various accompanying forceps.

ANESTHESIA

The Wigand total sphenoethmoidectomy can be performed under local or general anesthesia. We prefer general anesthesia because of the extensive nature of the procedure and to avoid aspiration from posterior nasal bleeding. However, in selected patients, the combination of infiltrative anesthesia and a sphenopalatine block via the greater palatine foramen is acceptable. In all cases, before prepping and draping the patient, the lateral wall of the nose, middle turbinate, and face of the sphenoid are injected with 1% lidocaine with 1:100,000 epinephrine. Before this, the nose is sprayed with Afrin or an equivalent vasoconstrictive agent and packed with gauze saturated with a similar solution. If a septoplasty is indicated for either airway obstruction or accessibility to the posterior paranasal sinuses, the septum also is injected at this time. On an average, 20 ml to 25 ml of 1% lidocaine with 1:100,000 epinephrine is used for bilateral procedures and septoplasty. After completing injection of the nose, the vasoconstrictive agent-saturated packing is replaced in the nasal cavity. The patient is then prepped and draped for surgery so that the sterile field includes superiorly the brow and inferiorly the upper lip. When general endotracheal anesthesia is used, a sterile plastic drape may be placed over the upper lip and chin to permit visualization of the endotracheal tube, thus monitoring the airway.

SURGICAL PROCEDURE

Step 1   (Illustrated on pages 108–109)

When indicated, a septoplasty is performed before beginning endoscopic sinus surgery. The nose is examined with an appropriate endoscope (25-degree or 30-degree wide-angle telescope or standard 0-degree and 30-degree telescopes) (Figure 6.2). Care should be taken to clearly discern the middle turbinate, the ostiomeatal complex, the anterior wall of the sphenoid sinus, and the lateral wall of the nose.

Step 2   (Illustrated on pages 110–111)

The inferior aspect of the middle turbinate is transected with two incisions using turbinate scissors. The first incision is parallel to the inferior free margin of the turbinate and removes approximately the inferior one third of this structure. The second incision begins at the midportion in an anterior-posterior direction of the turbinate and is directed posteriorly and superiorly toward the upper aspect of the anterior wall of the sphenoid sinus. This second incision results in a partial opening into the posterior ethmoid cells (Figures 6.3). This step can be modified to include only the posterior incision and thus preserve the entire anterior portion of the middle turbinate (Figure 6.3C).

Step 3 (Illustrated on pages 112–113)

Depending on the visualization of the sphenoid ostium, either this structure may be identified as lying at approximately the same level as the posterior insertion of the middle turbinate and the superior turbinate, or it may be necessary to remove further posterior ethmoid cells (Figure 6.4). In the latter case, 45-degree Weil-Blakesley ethmoid forceps are used for this purpose (Figure 6.4B). The endoscope should be positioned so as to permit full visualization of every aspect of the entire surgical procedure. In locating the sphenoid ostium, the physician should recall that this structure is approximately 7 cm from the maxillary spine at an angle of 30 degrees from the nasal floor. This ostium may be confirmed by using either a calibrated probe, such as a Cottle elevator, or rigid suction. Punch forceps are used to remove the anterior wall of the sphenoid sinus inferior to the ostium of this cavity (Figure 6.4D). The sinus is then examined endoscopically, and biopsies are taken as necessary. The convexity formed by the internal carotid artery can be visualized in the lateral wall of the sphenoid sinus, as can in some cases the optic nerve in the superior lateral aspect of the sphenoid sinus.

Step 4 (Illustrated on pages 114–115)

After completion of the sphenoidotomy, the posterior ethmoid cells are reentered and exenterated using the combination of the 45- and 90-degree Weil-Blakesley ethmoid forceps (Figure 6.5). Care is taken to identify the fovea ethmoidalis, which serves as the superior boundary of the dissection (Figure 6.5A). This landmark should be identified throughout the rest of the procedure. While visualizing the fovea ethmoidalis, the anterior ethmoid cells are exenterated. The anterior limit of this procedure is reached when the frontal recess cells of the ethmoid are removed and the ostium or nasofrontal duct is identified (Figure 6.5D).

Step 5 (Illustrated on pages 116–119)

The ostium, or duct of the frontal sinus, is inspected for patency (Figures 6.6, 6.7). All frontal recess cells are carefully removed from this site so as to preclude postsurgical obstruction of the outflow of the frontal sinus. The ostium or duct of this sinus is not entered unless there is radiographic evidence of frontal sinusitis, and, in fact, in many individuals the removal of the frontal recess cells may be sufficient to resolve recurrent frontal sinusitis.

This passage may be cannulated with curved suction, and inspissated secretions may be removed. If the outflow of the frontal sinus is obstructed or tissue must be removed from this sinus, the anterior wall of the ostium or duct can be removed partially using either punch forceps or diamond burr. Using the appropriate endoscope (wide-angle 70-degree telescope or standard 90-degree and 120-degree telescopes), the frontal sinus can be examined. The various angled double spoon forceps are useful for removing lesions within the frontal sinus (Figure 6.6D). By resecting the agger nasi cells, the frontal recess cells and ostium or duct of the frontal sinus are better visualized (Figures 6.6A, B, C, 6.7A). As a generality, when a 4 mm suction probe can be easily passed into the frontal sinus, good healing of this passage can be expected.

Step 6 (Illustrated on pages 120–123)

The placement of a supra-inferior turbinate antrostomy can be performed either at the beginning or at the end of this technique (Figure 6.8). Usually, it is beneficial to perform this at the beginning if the ostium of the maxillary sinus can be clearly identified, and the retrograde forceps are used to enlarge this ostium. In many patients, this is not the case, and the antrostomy is performed as the last procedure. This step is begun by using either a 45-degree or 90-degree Weil-Blakesley forceps placed immediately above the superior surface of the inferior turbinate and directed in a strictly inferolateral direction (Figure 6.8E). In many patients, this aspect of the lateral wall of the nose is membranous and can be distinguished from the adjacent bone by palpation. After the forceps have entered the maxillary sinus, they may be opened and withdrawn to force the mucous membrane of the medial aspect of the antrum into the nose and to permit its removal. The Weil-Blakesley forceps and retrograde forceps are useful to enlarge the antrostomy to approximately 1.5 to 2 cm (Figure 6.8D). This entire maneuver must be performed with great care to avoid injury to the adjacent orbit. The maxillary sinus is inspected with the more acutely angled endoscopes (wide-angle 70-degree telescope or standard 70-degree and 120-degree telescopes), and tissue may be removed using the double spoon forceps (Figure 6.8A, B).

Step 7

The last step consists of inspection of the entire operative field for residual fragments of bone and mucous membrane. It is important to remove these, since they may either obstruct the outflow of the sinuses or form a later nidus for infection. The nasal cavity may then be irrigated with normal saline, and hemostasis may be obtained with cautery. If a septoplasty has been performed, the application of septal splints between the septum and middle turbinate is recommended. Packing should be kept at a minimum and may, in most people, consist of instilling antibiotic ointment under endoscopic visualization within the actual sinus cavities.

Figure 6.2. Step 1.

6.2A

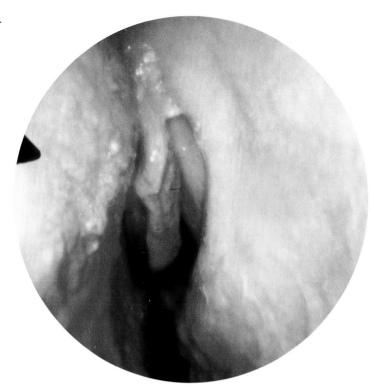

Figure 6.2A. After injection of a local anesthetic for hemostasis, the first step of the Wigand procedure is to inspect the entire nasal cavity. This endoscopic photograph of the left nose is typical of findings in the normal nose as seen by a 25-degree wide-angle telescope held in the anterior nasal cavity.

Figure 6.2B. Artist's illustration of Figure 6.2A shows middle turbinate, unicate process, bulla ethmoidalis, and nasal septum.

Figure 6.2C. This parasagittal section shows the anatomy of the lateral nasal wall, frontal sinus, sphenoid sinus, nasopharynx, and pituitary gland. The endoscope should be passed along the floor of the nose to the nasopharynx, and the anatomy of the nasopharynx, middle turbinate and inferior lateral nasal wall should be inspected. The second passage of the endoscope should seek to visualize the middle meatus and, when possible, the ostium of the sphenoid sinus. The last passage of the endoscope should be for the purpose of examining as well as possible the frontal recess region.

6.2B

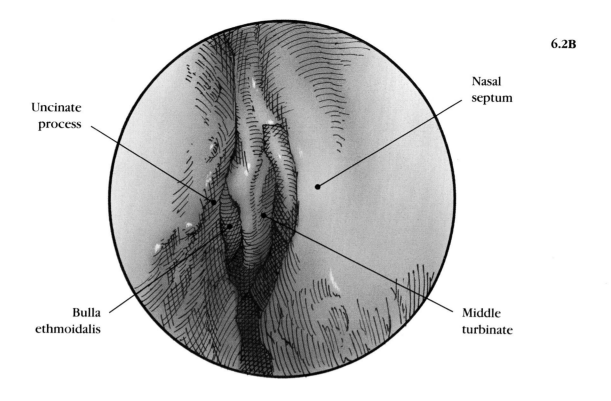

Uncinate process

Nasal septum

Bulla ethmoidalis

Middle turbinate

6.2C

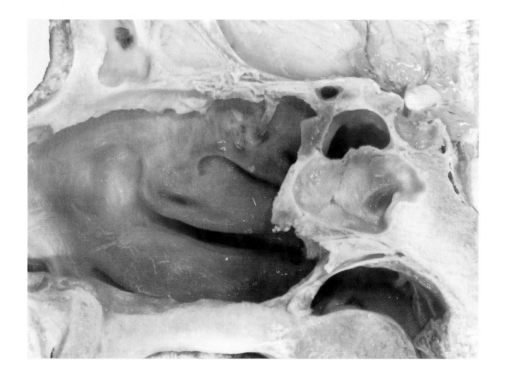

Figure 6.3. Step 2.

6.3A

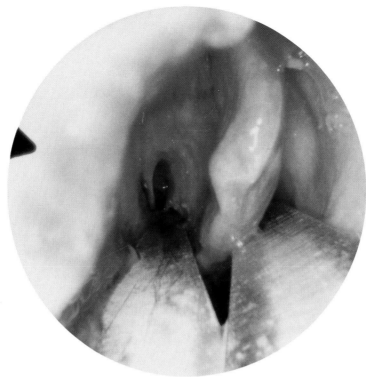

Figure 6.3A The inferior aspect of the middle turbinate is transected using turbinate scissors.

Figure 6.3B. Artist's illustration of Figure 6.3A showing transection of the posterior aspect of the middle turbinate. Note ostium of sphenoid sinus posteriorly.

Figure 6.3C. As originally described, the Wigand technique includes partial transection of the inferior aspect of the middle turbinate. The procedure can be modified as is shown in the sagittal dissection to consist solely of resection of the posterior portion of this turbinate.

6.3B

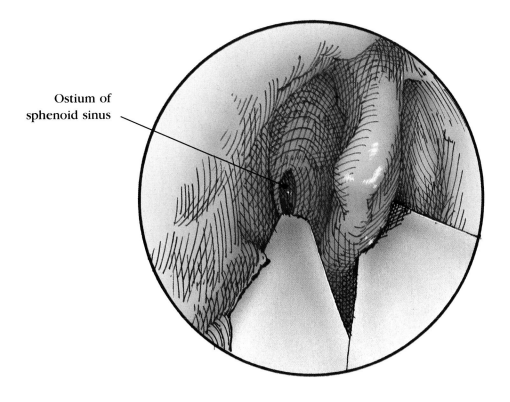

Ostium of
sphenoid sinus

6.3C

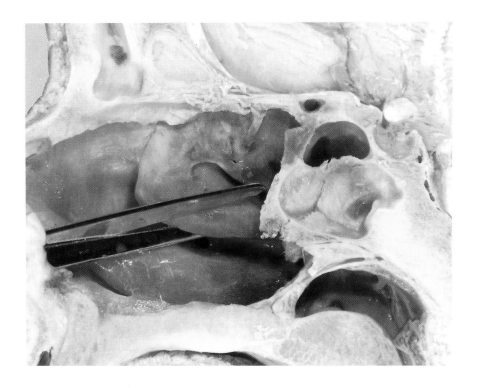

Figure 6.4. Step 3.

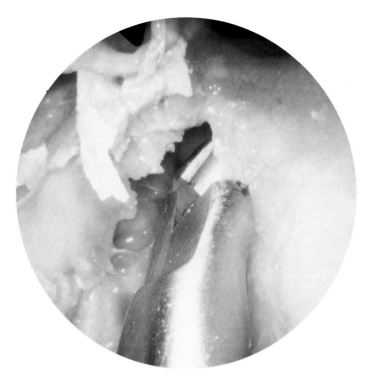

Figure 6.4A. The ostium of the sphenoid sinus is exposed by partial resection of the middle turbinate and enlarged using punch forceps. In many subjects, as was shown in Figure 6.3, the ostium of the sphenoid sinus is readily identifiable without transection of the turbinate. In some cases, identification of the ostium is aided by using either a rigid suction or a calibrated probe to cannulate the sinus.

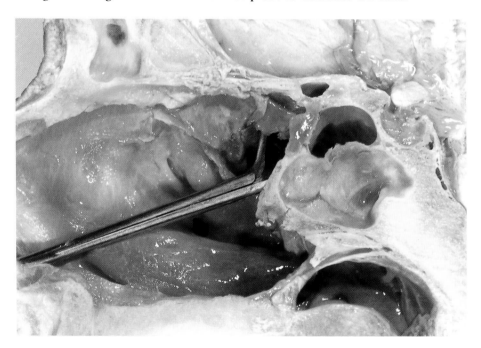

Figure 6.4B. In a significant number of people, the sphenoid ostium is still not visible after transection of the posterior aspect of the middle turbinate. In these patients, it is necessary to remove several of the posterior ethmoid cells to better visualize the anterior wall of the sphenoid sinus.

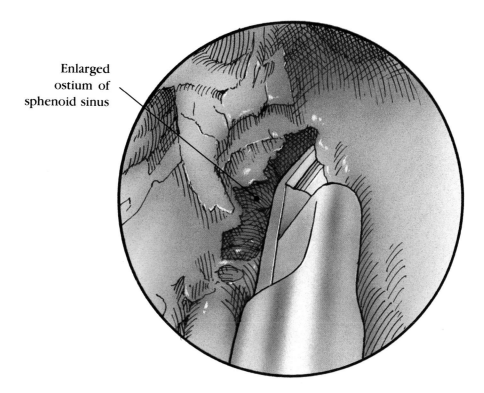

Enlarged ostium of sphenoid sinus

Figure 6.4C. Artist's illustration shows punch forceps enlarging sphenoid ostium.

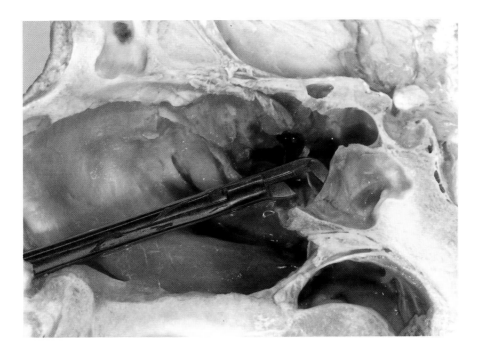

Figure 6.4D. After the ostium of the sphenoid sinus is enlarged, the inferior and medial aspects of the anterior wall can be safely removed. The lateral aspect of the anterior wall of the sphenoid sinus should be removed with great care to avoid potential injury to the internal carotid artery and optic nerve. The sinus is then carefully inspected, and under direct vision, biopsies are taken.

Figure 6.5. Step 4.

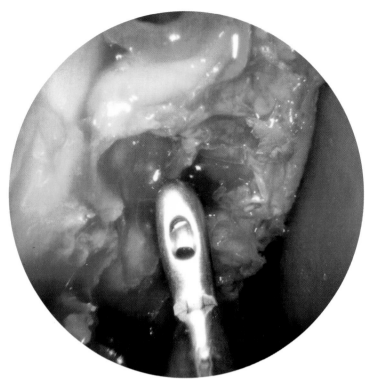

Figure 6.5A. After completion of the sphenoidotomy, the posterior ethmoids are reentered and exenterated. The fovea ethmoidalis forms the superior boundary of the dissection.

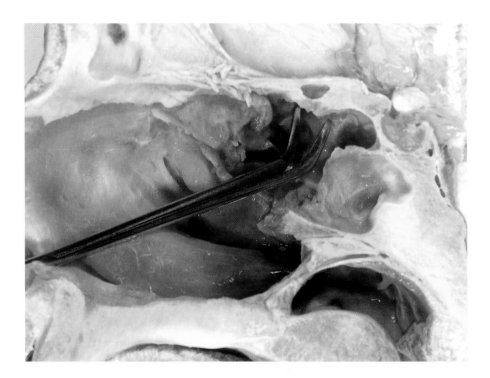

Figure 6.5B. Weil-Blakesley forceps are shown in the posterior ethmoid sinus. Note that the tip of the forceps is against the fovea ethmoidalis at the junction of the posterior ethmoids and sphenoid sinus.

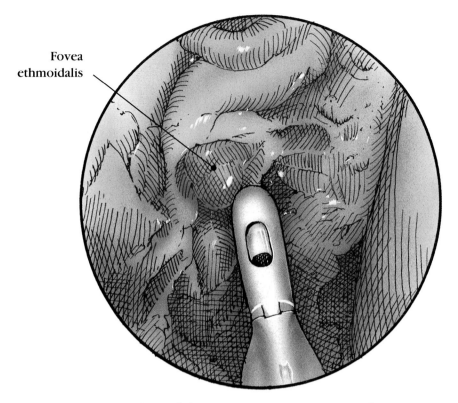

Fovea
ethmoidalis

Figure 6.5C. Artist's illustration of Figure 6.5A.

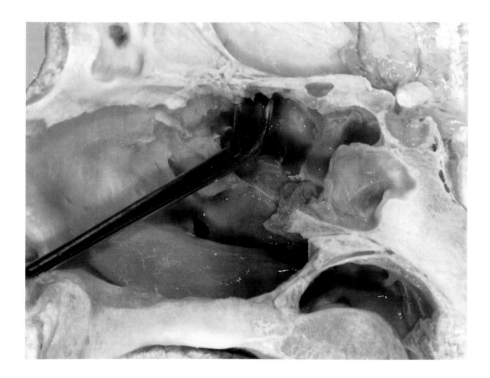

Figure 6.5D. While visualizing the fovea, the dissection proceeds anteriorly until all the ethmoid cells are removed.

Figure 6.6. Step 5.

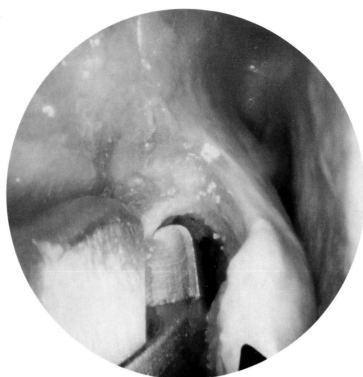

Figure 6.6A. The anterior limit of the procedure is exenteration of the frontal recess cells of the ethmoid. Visualization of the entire frontal recess is greatly facilitated if the agger nasi cells are partially removed with a punch or Weil-Blakesley forceps.

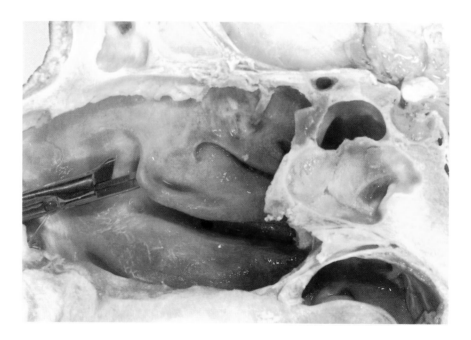

Figure 6.6B. The position of the forceps is shown as it would normally appear before transection of the turbinate or removal of this structure, as has been necessary for demonstration of the procedure in previous figures.

116

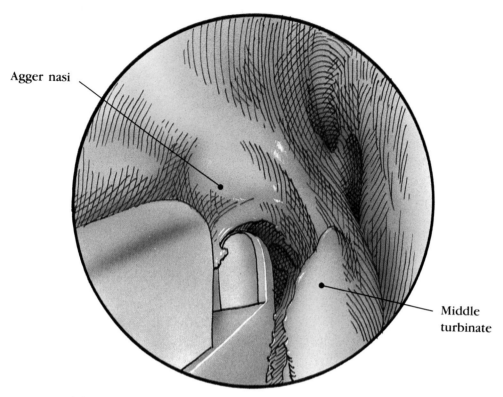

Agger nasi

Middle
turbinate

Figure 6.6C. Artist's illustration shows resection of agger nasi cells, with frontal recess posterior and frontal sinus posteriosuperior to these cells.

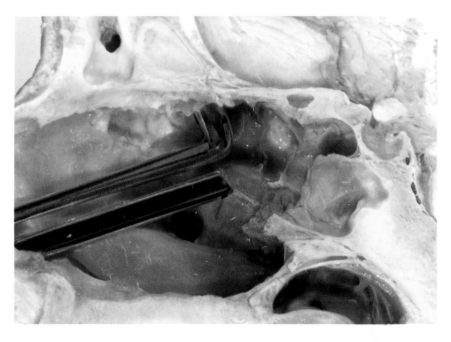

Figure 6.6D. Anterior ethmoid cells are removed to gain further access to frontal recess cells using 90-degree Weil-Blakesley and double spoon forceps.

Figure 6.7. Step 5 (continued).
6.7A

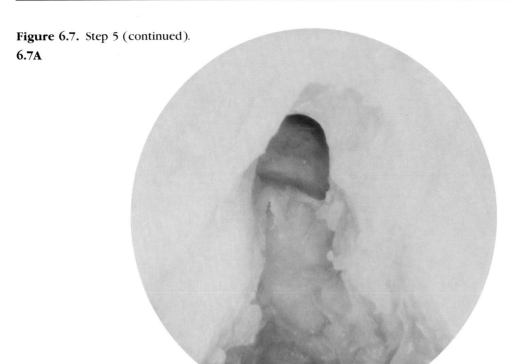

Figure 6.7A. Frontal recess is carefully cleaned of diseased mucous membrane, and the nasofrontal duct or ostium is entered only if the frontal sinus is abnormal. As is shown, the frontal sinus can be visualized satisfactorily using either standard 90-degree and 120-degree telescopes or wide-angle 70-degree telescope.

Figure 6.7B. Note in this artist's illustration of Figure 6.7A, the posterior wall of the frontal sinus as seen after removal of the frontal recess cells.

Figure 6.7C. As demonstrated, double spoon forceps can be placed within the frontal recess and frontal sinus to remove diseased tissue under direct observation using angled telescopes.

6.7B

Posterior wall of
frontal sinus

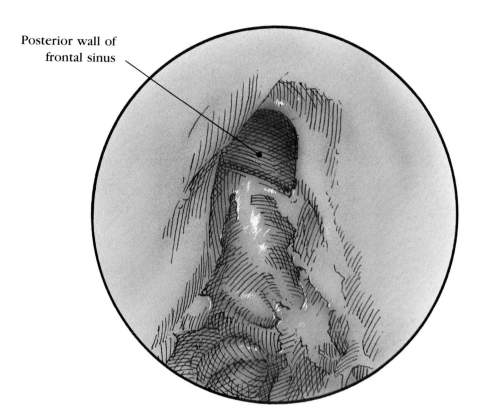

6.7C

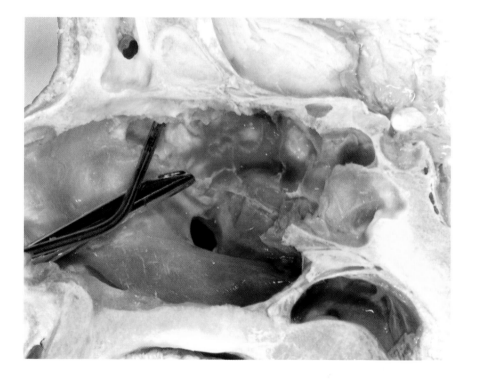

Figure 6.8. Step 6.

6.8A

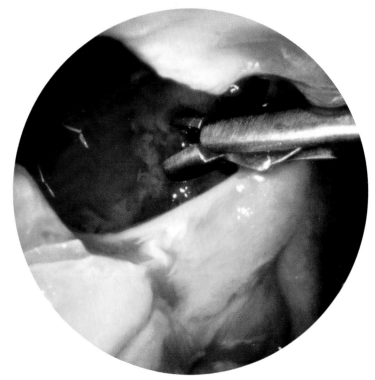

Figure 6.8A. Double spoon forceps are shown biopsying the posterior lateral wall of the maxillary sinus after performing a supra-inferior turbinate antrostomy.

Figure 6.8B. Artist's illustration of Figure 6.8A.

Figure 6.8C. Double spoon forceps are seen entering the antrostomy while being viewed through an angled telescope.

Figures 6.8D and **68E** on pages 122 and 123.

6.8B

Posterior wall of
maxillary sinus

Inferior
turbinate

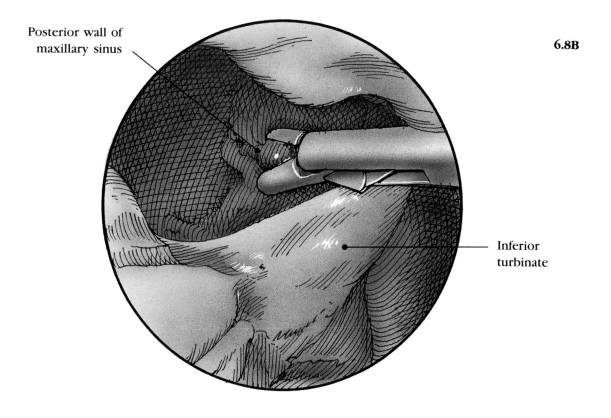

6.8C

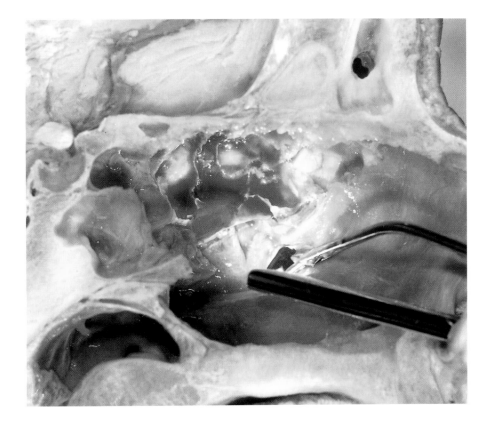

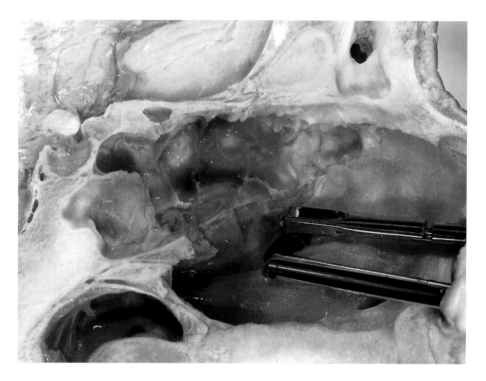

Figure 6.8D. The antrostomy can be formed by using two different techniques or a combination of both of these methods. First, when the natural ostium of the maxillary sinus can be identified, the retrograde forceps, as are shown, may be used to enlarge this ostium anteriorly.

HIGHLIGHTS

1. Total sphenoethmoidectomy is designed to eliminate the need for other more invasive procedures, such as Caldwell-Luc, transantral or external ethmoidectomy, and osteoplastic flap with fat obliteration, in the majority of patients with extensive paranasal sinus disease.

2. As in all endoscopic paranasal sinus surgery, the eyes must be included in the sterile field and monitored closely.

3. Resection of the agger nasi cells is most useful in permitting inspection of the ostium or duct of the frontal sinus.

4. Gross polyps can be removed using a headlight, before injection of local anesthetic, to permit accurate placement of the anesthetic agent.

POSTOPERATIVE CARE

The patient is given an instruction sheet before surgery that outlines those activities to be performed and avoided. The most important of these is irrigation of the nose with normal saline on the second postoperative day. This is best accomplished using a nasal irrigation attachment for the Water Pik. Saline can either be purchased by the liter or made by having the patient use 2 cups of boiled water for every teaspoon of salt. The patient is in-

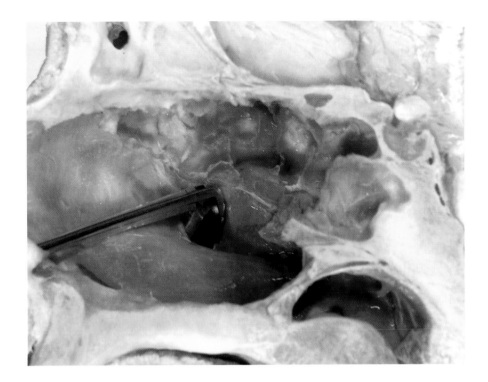

Figure 6.8E. When the ostium of the maxillary sinus is not visible, the 90-degree Weil-Blakesley forceps can be placed through the membranous meatus region of the maxillary sinus. These forceps, or the retrograde forceps, can be used to enlarge the ostium to approximately 1.5 to 2 cm in diameter. Completing inspection of the maxillary sinus requires the use of either a standard 120-degree or a 70-degree wide-angle telescope. The procedure is now complete, and the nose should be inspected for residual hemorrhage, and appropriate packing should be placed.

structed to irrigate a minimum of 1 cup of saline (or until the effluent from the nose is clear) three times a day for the first 3 weeks. The patient is encouraged thereafter to irrigate their nose indefinitely at least once a day.

Postoperative visits begin on the second through fourth day. The nose is carefully cleaned of dried secretions and blood approximately twice a week for the first 3 weeks. Once the operative field has been covered by mucous membrane, office visits are less frequent. However, patients are encouraged to maintain periodic visits in the hope of recognizing and correcting early recurrent disease.

Nasal steroids are begun by the end of the first postoperative week, while antibiotics are discontinued by the fifth postoperative day. In the nonallergic patient without polyps and without other contraindications, such as pregnancy, these medications are used for approximately 6 months. In the allergic or polyp patient, nasal steroids form an important, long-term adjuvant to the medical and surgical management.

COMPLICATIONS

The two major potential complications of endoscopic total sphenoethmoidectomy are the same as those with conventional approaches to the sinuses, injury to the eye and brain.

Ophthalmologic Injuries

During the performance of either the ethmoidectomy or the antrostomy, the lamina papyracea can be perforated and the orbital tissues injured. The most common of these injuries is disruption of the orbital fat and hemorrhage. In a minor compromise of these structures, the outcome will be only ecchymosis in the medial canthal region. With greater trauma, orbital hematoma may occur, and immediate confirmation by CT or MR imaging, followed by drainage, is recommended. Less common is partial or complete transection of the medial rectus or superior oblique muscles. The least common injury is trauma to the optic nerve. In the normal patient, the optic nerve is surrounded by dense bone, and if the surgeon follows the rule of avoiding the removal of such bone, injury is unlikely. In the rare patient, the optic canal may be partially dehiscent, exposing the nerve in either the sphenoid or posterior ethmoids. Such unusual events point out the need always to visualize well any area within the sinuses before removing tissue. Occasionally, this may be anticipated on preoperative CT scanning.

Neurologic Injuries

The most common neurologic complication of sinus surgery is cerebrospinal fluid fistula. This tends to result from either avulsion of the olfactory filia, penetration of the fovea ethmoidalis, or fracture of the bony plate. The first problem can be avoided by remaining lateral to the middle turbinate during surgery. The second cause of cerebrospinal fluid fistula is best prevented by painstaking visualization of the fovea. The last chance of this complication is the inadvertent torquing of the fovea during the removal of the ethmoid labyrinth.

Whatever the cause, minor injuries can be repaired intraoperatively using tissue glues and fascial or muscle grafts applied under endoscopic control. In such cases, a spinal drain is particularly useful in controlling the fistula. The other major, and fortunately seldom seen, neurologic complication is laceration of the internal carotid artery. This vessel is most vulnerable, since it impinges on the lateral wall of the sphenoid sinus and, like the optic nerve, the bony covering of the artery may be dehiscent. The need for careful visualization of the lateral wall of the sphenoid is obvious.

LITERATURE CITED

Wigand, M. E.
  1981 Transnasal ethmoidectomy under endoscopical control. *Rhinology*, 19:7–12.
Wigand, M. E., Steiner, W., and Jaumann, M. P.
  1978 Endonasal sinus surgery with endoscopical control: From radical operation to rehabilitation of the mucosa. *Endoscopy*, 10:255–260.

Index

Index entries for figures and tables are indicated by italicized numbers.